T0130654

Cancer: the key to getting the best care
Making the system work for you

Advance Acclaim by senior doctors:

Cancer: the key to getting the best care

Making the system work for you

Professor Karol Sikora

MA, MD, PhD, FRCR, FRCP, FFPM

Professor of Cancer Medicine and Consultant Oncologist; Founding Dean, University of Buckingham Medical School; Former Chief WHO Cancer Programme, Geneva; Former Chairman, Department of Cancer Medicine, Imperial College, Hammersmith Hospital, London

EER

Edward Everett Root. Brighton. 2023

EER

Edward Everett Root, Publishers, Co. Ltd., Atlas Chambers,
33 West Street, Brighton, Sussex, BN1 2RE, England.
*Full details of our stock-holding overseas agents in America, Australia, China,
Europe and Japan, and how to order our books, are given on our website.*

www.eerpublishing.com

edwardeverettroot@yahoo.co.uk

We Stand With Ukraine!
EER books are **NOT** available for sale in Russia or Belarus.

Karol Sikora © 2023
Cancer: the key to getting the best care
Making the system work for you

ISBN: 978-1-915115-17-1 Hardback
ISBN: 978-1-915115-18-8 Paperback
ISBN: 978-1-915115-19-5 eBook

Design and production by Pageset Ltd., High Wycombe, Buckinghamshire.

About the author

Professor Karol Sikora is a leading consultant oncologist in the UK. He studied medicine at Corpus Christi College, Cambridge where he obtained a double first. His clinical training was at Middlesex Hospital where he earned distinctions in medicine, clinical pharmacology and obstetrics. After junior doctor posts in London and Cambridge he began his career in cancer medicine as a registrar at St Bartholomew's Hospital. He became an MRC Research Fellow at the Laboratory for Molecular Biology in Cambridge where he completed a PhD supervised by Nobel Laureate, Sydney Brenner. He then spent nearly two years as a Clinical Fellow in cancer medicine at Stanford University Hospital, California before returning to direct the Ludwig Institute for Cancer Research at Cambridge. In 1986, he was appointed Professor and Chairman of the Department of Cancer Medicine at Hammersmith Hospital, London which subsequently became part of Imperial College School of Medicine. He was seconded to be Director of the World Health Organisation, Cancer Programme in Geneva and Lyon from 1999–2000. He is still an honorary Consultant Oncologist at Hammersmith.

He became adviser on cancer to HCA hospitals internationally. He subsequently created Cancer Partners UK – Britain's largest independent cancer network of ten centres, funded by private equity with significant numbers of NHS patients under contract. This was subsequently integrated into Genesis Care. In 2015, he created and became medical director of Rutherford Health which has built four cancer centres with proton beam capability. He also was the joint founder of cancer centres in Nassau, Bahamas Providenciales, Turks and Caicos and St Johns, Antigua. He is currently the senior medical advisor to the Gulf International Cancer Centre, Abu Dhabi.

He was the Founding Dean and Professor of Medicine at Britain's first independent Medical School at the University of Buckingham. The school opened in 2015 with 67 students and now has a yearly intake of over 200 using local hospitals for their clinical training. A second campus has opened in Crewe to meet demand. He was recently a member of the Trust Board of Buckinghamshire Hospitals for 3 years and chaired the Partnership of East London Cooperatives (PELC) which includes NHS111, urgent care and out of hours GP services for a large part of East London.

He has published over 300 papers and written or edited 20 books including *Treatment of Cancer* – the standard British postgraduate textbook, now in its seventh edition in over 30 years. His previous book published by Edward Everett Root Publishers was *The Street-wise Patients Guide to Surviving Cancer*, issued in 2016 and widely used by cancer patients and their families.

He was made a Life Fellow of Corpus Christi College, Cambridge. During the Covid crisis he joined Twitter and now has over 300,000 followers and has been dubbed the *Positive Professor*. He is married with three children and six grandchildren. He enjoys long distance walking and old railways. Every Christmas he spends weekends as Father Christmas on a local heritage steam train.

Contents

Preface

It's a Monday morning in a busy oncology clinic in West London. There are two patients anxiously waiting to be seen for the first time. One is informed, pleasant, full of interesting questions and is chatting to the receptionist about her children. The other is grumpy, complaining about the ten-minute delay and the lack of coffee and has not made any effort to research the treatments likely to be advised. One will sail through their treatment keeping all the hospital staff cheerfully on their side. The other will be what we call in the trade – 'a heartsink patient' – someone to be avoided. Which would you rather be and who will have a better chance of beating the system?

Every health system is intimidating and the British one especially so. The language, the information gap between the patient and their health professionals, the mystique of medicine and the massive number of cancer information sites on the web will seem almost impenetrable especially as a diagnosis of cancer may have come as a major shock.

The other peculiar thing in Britain is that many people treat our National Health Service (NHS) as some sort of religion. They think it's a holy shrine – a force of good in a bad and dysfunctional world. Those that dare to criticize it as a bureaucratic monster with an appalling record of customer service are branded as heretics. I once said on BBC Newsnight that 'the NHS was the last bastion of communism in Europe'. I've never been forgiven for that. But where else in a consumer-driven world would you have to wait at least four hours to be seen in an emergency room, over a year to get a hip replacement or must beg with a grumpy receptionist to get an in-person appointment with a GP having first waited over half an hour for her to answer the phone? In any other service culture, you would just go somewhere else. That of course is the problem. You have no other place to go. Like any massive organization – by far the biggest employer in Britain – it is impossible to understand. I've worked in it for over 50 years. In this book you will get tips about how to use it to your advantage for your loved ones or yourself. And of course, and most importantly, how to get yourself to the top of the queue.

And here lies a moral point – should you do this? After all others may wait longer because of your success. In 1985, a British Airtours (part of British Airways) plane caught fire on take-off from Manchester Airport. 55 people died mainly in the back of the plane. The exception was a young man in seat 20B. Everyone else in the rear rows was quickly incapacitated by the toxic fumes and died. The only explanation is that he was so driven to survive that he jumped over many in front of him to reach the exit. Ethicists can debate forever whether this was reasonable – but maybe if you've been trapped in the NHS cancer maze, you just need to put yourself first if you want to survive. Remember seat 20B – I will refer to it frequently.

Sometimes it's worth paying to unblock any delay. Private hospitals are notoriously opaque about their charges. But it's easy to shop around for the cost of a CT or MRI scan which can often be done tomorrow for around £300. Unless you have private insurance or are very well heeled, it's best to use the NHS for your main cancer treatments. After all you've paid the price for them already in your taxes. I will explain how to sort things out. As you will see some of the new cancer drug schedules would set you back over £200,000 for a year's treatment.

I've tried to make this book as jargon-free, practical, and informative as possible. It explains how best to survive with a potentially life-threatening illness. It's often difficult to always act positively and get the best possible care when confronted with cancer. When should you push for results, information and help and when should you just trust the system, relax, and hope for the best?

The cancer system is just like the maze on the front cover of this book. The minute you are told you have cancer you are trapped in it. There are many routes to choose, a lot of blind alleys and not necessarily a clear way out. Once you understand the system and how it works you can determine the best way to get back to normal – physically, mentally, and spiritually. This book will help you work the system to your advantage.

I've been a cancer specialist and a consultant in Britain's NHS for 42 years.

Drawing on this extensive experience this book provides practical advice on how to make sure of the precise diagnosis and get the best treatment options. It will show you how to unblock delays and get results you've been promised but not delivered. The system is creaking with politicians promising the earth but unable to reform the monolith of the NHS. And its high priests are full of reassuring statements to the press about billions being poured in to improve services, how it has a superb learning culture from its mistakes and that it's really not too bad at all. But just don't believe them. Curiously, they all have private medical insurance.

Reading this I hope will help you to become an informed, positive, successful and above all a welcomed patient and yet make the system work for you.

Chapter One: your battle against cancer

Facing the news, taking control and making the system work for you

It may well be the worst news that you will hear in your whole life so far. You'll be sitting in a room, facing a person you hardly know – indeed you may never have met them before. You might well have a husband or wife or partner there with you, or a son or daughter, but you might well be alone. You'll be in a strange place. You may already be feeling unwell, otherwise you wouldn't be there, and you'll also be feeling very anxious about what lies ahead.

The news is not good. You have cancer.

Even before you step into the room to see your doctor, you should ask yourself this simple question. How do I feel about this?

For many people, when they are told that they have cancer, it will be the first time that they have confronted their own mortality. Of course, they will have known that they were going to die one day. We all do. But it is probably not something they have thought about much. They won't have reckoned on it happening to them, at least not this soon. Death will have been something that happened to other people, or far in the future, after their children and perhaps grandchildren were all grown up. It won't have been something they were reckoning on having to deal with right here and right now.

Now it is staring them in the face.

In my long experience as a cancer specialist, I have discovered that there are as many different reactions to the news as there are different types of people. Some people go to pieces. Some people go into a deep silent depression. Some start to get busy, treating their cancer as a task to be organised, managed, and dealt with rather like a business project. A few go into denial and try to pretend it just isn't happening to them, or that it will all go away in the morning when they wake up to a new day.

Whatever type of reaction you have – and there is no right or wrong way to cope with the news that you have cancer – this book is about helping you through the next few months. And, with luck, it will help you do so as calmly, stoically, and as successfully as possible. It will also ensure you get the best treatment available, whatever type of healthcare system you are using.

Because whether you are hysterical or stoical won't in the end make very much difference at all. What patients need to do most of all is immediately to start taking back control of their own treatment. And this will mean learning a lot of new information – and about how a whole very convoluted industry works.

When you are told you have cancer, you are about to go into a system – the cancer industry. I don't mean to disparage the work of all the people within the system in the slightest. The doctors, nurses, other clinicians, health care managers and even drug company executives all mean well. They do the best they can for patients, often in very difficult and trying circumstances. Not all of them are angels. But few of them are devils either. Mostly they are a group of intelligent, hard-working people going about their work. Sure, there is conflict when the heady aspirations of business, greed, altruism and trying to get the best care possible for yourself collide.

You need to understand one very simple point. The system is not actually there to help you – or at least not you alone.

The system is there to help maximise the quality of cancer treatment overall, to make sure the organisation and the people within it make a living and to make sure the burden on society is not too great. Of course, much of the time that will mean treating your cancer as quickly and effectively as possible. But – and this is the important point – not all the time.

As a patient, you need to learn how the system works. And you need to learn how to make sure it works for you all the time.

With any luck, that is what this book will be able to do – teach you how the system works, from someone who has spent an entire career inside it and show you how you can make it work better for you. It doesn't matter whether you are rich or poor, black or white, or have been educated at university or not. Nor does it matter how the health system you are using works – tax based as in Britain or Canada; social insurance as in much of Europe, or a cut-throat free market economy as in the USA or many poorer countries. If you take charge of your own destiny, you will get the best treatment possible. If you don't, then you will be at the mercy of a system whatever it is.

The most important person is you – so you must be satisfied that you are getting the best treatment possible. Do not be put off by bureaucracy or complexity – you only get one bite at the cherry – you need to get the best type of treatment right from the start. Negotiate calmly without aggression and usually locked doors will simply open and a mutually satisfactory solution found.

That's why you need this book – because the later chapters will give you an insiders' guide to making sure you get the best treatment possible, regardless of cost. The next chapter gives you a summary of what cancer is and how it's treated. Obviously, it's not tailored to your problem or your country, but it will help you go to the web and find out more about exactly your problem. The internet if used correctly will act as your guide to the best treatment for you that's possible today.

I have spent most of my career in Britain where our great institution the NHS is viewed as a religion by many. What exasperates me is that although it can deliver world class cancer care for some people for many it is a very low-quality system where the five 'D's' of rationing dominate – delay, denial, deflection, discrimination and determination by committee. Let me give you a concrete example of how the system gets overridden by those in the know. These things go on in all countries and not just Britain.

Tony Blair was our prime minister in 2003 when he developed acute chest pain and a very rapid pulse at 2 pm on a beautiful summer Sunday afternoon. He was in the elegant mansion used by British leaders called Chequers, deep in the splendid Buckinghamshire countryside. The nearest hospital with a cardiac care facility was twenty miles away in Aylesbury. A cavalcade with a police escort set off immediately, with the local cardiologist summoned and taken by police car to the hospital.

But enquiries were made, and it was soon very clear that Aylesbury had no facilities for emergency stenting – which just means putting a tube directly into the coronary arteries to unblock them immediately after a heart attack. After a series of terse telephone calls the whole high-speed procession carried on past Aylesbury and drove at an even faster pace a further thirty miles down the motorway to Hammersmith Hospital in West London. This houses one of Britain's leading heart centres and provides a 24-hour immediate stenting service. I was head of cancer medicine at the time so got the whole story first-hand the next day from my friends in cardiology. It all turned out to be a false alarm. He had probably just drunk too much coffee, and this had triggered a relatively harmless abnormal rhythm called atrial fibrillation in his heart.

The point of this story is that if it were you with chest pain and the nice emergency ambulance crew were hurtling towards Aylesbury would you be well enough informed to get to Hammersmith? It could mean the difference between your life and death. And how could you get reliable information? Less than 70% of hospitals with emergency departments in Britain can perform immediate coronary stenting, especially at weekends. They don't advertise the fact – there's no publicly available database. The ambulance service can only take you to the nearest hospital with an emergency department. This is a great example of inequity and randomness in care. It happens all over the world. If you know about it you can act, but if you don't, you just must go with the flow. In this sort of situation, you have no time to control your journey but with cancer you do.

I was sixteen when my father Witold Sikora died from lung cancer. He had come across to Britain from Poland as a Captain in the Polish Army during World War II. He joined the signals regiment of the British Army located in Scotland. After the war ended my father made his career as an electrical engineer. He met my mother at an officer's dance in Edinburgh one Saturday night in 1944. She went with her sister – their parents must have been horrified or more likely they never knew. My mother was a Scottish school teacher. She valued education beyond everything. When she was 17, she had obtained a place at Edinburgh University to read chemistry, one of the very few women to do so at that time. But her parents were poor – my grandfather was the village butcher in Polmont. So, she had to forgo the place and go to teacher training college in Edinburgh instead as she could obtain government funding.

The combination of my father's typical immigrant ambition for me and my mother's determination that I would succeed were powerful drivers to the young Karol Sikora. I was an only child, so I had their undivided attention – not always welcome. My father dragged me round Oxford and Cambridge when I was ten and told me I had to go to one of these leading Universities. I vividly remember him saying that I could be a dustman afterwards, but I just had to get there first. Garbage collectors were obviously at the bottom of the social pile in Poland before the war.

My father died at the Royal Brompton Hospital in London from widespread lung cancer in his bones, kidneys, liver, and spleen. I was 16 at the time and it made a vivid impression. The specialists treating him didn't tell him or us what he was suffering from until the last possible moment. In those days, doctors told their patients as little as possible. My mother and I only found out that my father had lung cancer, and that he was not likely to recover, the day before he died. There was nothing unusual or cruel about the doctors treating my father, however. In those days, doctors always told their patients as little as possible – it was simply the way they worked. The view was that it was better for the patient not to know, and their families as well. There was nothing that they could do about it anyway, and the news would only upset them.

The week before he died my acceptance letter from Cambridge dropped through the letter box. I still remember the smile on his face when I told him my fantastic news.

We were far from alone in experiencing medical secrecy. Doctors routinely kept a patient's condition secret from them. One famous example was Eva Peron, the wildly popular wife of the Argentinian President Juan Peron. Eva suffered from cervical cancer (cancer of the neck of the womb), from which she died at the age of 33 in 1952. But her condition was never revealed to the public. Indeed, the American surgeon who treated her, George Pack, was flown into the country in complete secrecy, operating on her in the middle of the night, and then flew back to New York immediately. She never even saw him before or after the operation. Certainly, when she collapsed in public from profound anaemia, no one was told what the matter was. It was kept hidden from the public, just as much as her condition was kept secret from her.

Watch the film *Evita* with Madonna in the title part. It portrays the situation of the time extremely well. The lyrics of Andrew Lloyd-Weber's musical are revealing.

President Peron, Evita's husband, sings:

Your little body's slowly breaking down.
Your losing speed, your losing strength – not style – that goes on flourishing forever, but your eyes, your smile do not have the sparkle of your fantastic past.
If you climb one more mountain, it could be your last.

In reality, she had become profoundly anaemic because of her undiagnosed cancer.

Cancer was just not something people talked about until 25 years ago. It was practically a secret, a strange condition that only a few specialists in the medical profession knew anything about. I vividly remember going on ward rounds as a medical student where codes for cancer – mitotic activity, NG meaning new growth or neoplasia were used. Now we're much more upfront but still retreat behind a cloak of secrecy unless pushed for disclosure.

The relationship between doctors and their patients was very different to what it is today. But it still has a long way to go. The doctor and the rest of the health care system are a partner, but they are not in charge of your cancer. *You* are always in charge of it. Never forget this. Doctors and systems will be there long after you are gone. Use them to help you get the best care possible today.

After my father died, I wanted to know as much about cancer as possible – perhaps because the doctors had told us so little. My mother, like most women with a single son, was fiercely ambitious for me. She kept my nose to the grindstone all through school – it really wasn't much fun. It was annoying to me at the time. I would rather she had allowed me to spend more time messing around with my school friends and less swotting with my books. But looking back, I am grateful for her drive and her discipline. I got into Cambridge to read medicine, and it was from there that I could really start to learn about what cancer really was, where it had come from, and how we might start to go about treating it more effectively.

Before starting at Cambridge, I had six months to spend either at school or working as I was quite young for my year. I saw a job advertised as a laboratory technician at the Royal Marsden Hospital, a large specialist cancer hospital in London and applied – being completely honest about the short time I could spend. The consultant pathologist was amused by my ambition and said the job was mine for six months at the rather low salary of £50 a month. But it seemed like a fortune to me. It was really great fun working with some very interesting people and understanding what went on behind the scenes in a major cancer hospital. When I left, I was given a copy of *Gray's Anatomy* signed by everyone in the lab. I still have it and treasure it to this day.

Cambridge was a wonderful experience. I was at a small but beautiful college called Corpus Christi right in the centre nearly opposite the more famous King's College. I worked hard but also enjoyed a range of sports. As the smallest boy in the College, I was soon approached to be cox in the College boat. After a few bad accidents which involved crashing into a tree, another boat and causing mayhem at the Henley Regatta I calmed down and became cox of the College First Boat. It was increasingly difficult as a medical student to find time for serious rowing so in my last year I stopped. My mother kept nagging me about my work all the time.

I got a degree with very good marks – a double first in fact. For this I was thrown into the river by the Boat Club crew – in a typically good-natured way. I then went to London to do my clinical training at Middlesex Hospital, now part of University College Hospital London. I was so looking forward to my clinical training, but it was very poorly organized in those days. The first three months consisted of an introductory course. Endless repetition of what the Cambridge students thought was obvious. After this it got better but only because medicine wasn't really taught in those days, you just immersed yourself in it. 'See one, do one, teach one' was the mantra of medical education at the time. Whether it was taking a blood sample, putting in a chest drain or performing a lumbar puncture it was all the same.

Four months after starting my clinical course I found myself in a west London emergency department drinking coffee in the early morning hours of a Sunday morning when suddenly all hell broke loose. A major traffic accident had occurred on Western Avenue caused by a drunken driver. I'll never forget a young man who was gradually going blue despite being given oxygen by me. The registrar in charge who was busy amputating his girlfriend's leg in another cubicle yelled over to me to put in a chest drain. I'd no idea what he meant. In the end he came over swore at me and grabbed a plastic tube. He told me to stuff it in under the eighth rib and stitch it in place. Then he returned, still swearing under his breath, to his surgery. But my patient turned pink – we had saved him.

Three years of expensive education at Cambridge and it meant nothing in a practical way. But both patients survived. It taught me a real lesson. Only experience can really allow doctors to deliver first class care in whatever specialty they work.

After qualifying I worked as a houseman (now called a Foundation Doctor) for the Professor of Medicine at the Middlesex Hospital. It was great fun being a real doctor. I had a room in the hospital right in the heart of London and suddenly lots of girlfriends. But fate is strange. Our normal ward was being painted so I had patients all over the hospital. On one of our outlying wards, I met a very pretty blonde staff nurse called Alison on my very first day as a doctor. I remember she blushed when I met her as we had been on a ward together at one in the morning when I was a student a year back and I had botched putting up an intravenous drip on a patient. She had been very kind both to the poor patient and to me. I've now been married to her for nearly 50 years, and we have three grown up children and six grandchildren. Where would all of us be if the painters hadn't moved in?

I worked as a house surgeon at Cambridge with a very famous transplant pioneer, Professor Roy Calne. It was very challenging work and totally absorbing. In those days young doctors worked all hours but we were well looked after. In the summer I remember I worked for two weeks on call without ever leaving the hospital as my colleague was on holiday and there was no replacement. It wasn't really safe as on several occasions I was desperately tired.

After this I got a senior house officer job in cardiology at Hammersmith Hospital. This was a highly prestigious appointment as Hammersmith was the postgraduate medical school – a real centre of excellence. Cardiology was fascinating and pretty dramatic. Life and death went by on the ward. Sudden bad things happened – people's hearts sometimes stopped.

The lack of practicality of academic medicine was again forcibly rammed home one morning. I vividly remember having a coffee in the sister's office of Ward B2. Suddenly the hospital loudspeaker blared *"cardiac arrest ward B2"* three times. At that time there was no attempt to be a bit more subtle such as the US equivalent of *'code blue'* in public announcements. I rushed onto the ward to see where disaster had apparently struck but all was calm. I knew that one of the senior clinical research consultants who specialised on abnormal heart rhythms was on the ward. I quickly realised that he was behind the screens of bed 22 – exactly where the alarm had been sounded. I rushed in to find a nice old lady enjoying a cup of tea and the research physician blushing profusely. He was doing a clinical trial of a new heart drug and thought he had induced a cardiac arrest. He was reading the ECG trace without looking at the patient. The flat line he saw on the screen caused him to panic even though his patient was perfectly well. One of the electrodes had become disconnected so there was no signal. Within two minutes pandemonium erupted as the crash trolley and about ten people came rushing to join us. I told them politely to go away. Our patient wisely decided to have another cup of tea.

After Hammersmith, I became a temporary Casualty Officer for a month in Tunbridge Wells. Alison, my fiancé was a midwife at the local maternity unit so we could meet on our days off. Being at the front door of the hospital was fun and exciting especially after hours when nobody else was around. All sorts of people came by with problems for me to solve. There were serious accidents, minor injuries, heart attacks – everyday problems in an emergency department.

The most bizarre was a man who undressed himself in the bus station at teatime. Suddenly there were a lot of sirens. The naked man, now covered with blankets, was brought out of the ambulance by several burly policemen. I examined him and found nothing wrong. What was I supposed to do? Nothing in my training was relevant here so I had a quiet word with the Police Sergeant. Well Sir, he said politely, people just don't take their clothes off at the bus station – this is Tunbridge Wells after all. So, for the next three hours I went through the laborious process of sorting out his compulsory detention in a psychiatric hospital on the South Coast. His acute problem was handled well but once the excitement was over everybody disappeared leaving it to me. That's very relevant to everything we do in medicine and even in cancer.

This happened again to me even more dramatically a few months later. I was working as an on-call GP with a relief service in South London on my weekend off from the hospital. In those days these services had very few doctors covering an awful lot of patients. It was crazy – I was paid an hourly rate, but the driver was paid per visit. So, he was incentivized to drive fast and speed me up so I could do more calls. We had a crackly car radio – it was long before mobile phones.

One Sunday afternoon we had an urgent call to go to a pub at the Trafalgar Square end of Whitehall called the Silver Cross. It's still there – I had a beer there last week. The landlady had apparently been expressing suicidal ideas and was on the fifth floor sitting on the outside window ledge overlooking the road.

We arrived in twenty minutes. The scene looked like a film set. About a dozen policemen, two fire engines and an ambulance were in place. The road was blocked. Everyone was waiting for the doctor. I was 23 years old and had almost no psychiatric training. There was nothing in my books about how to handle this. I was treated like the great healer as I went into the pub. The landlord had clearly had a few drinks already and graciously offered me one which I wisely declined. We went up to the fifth floor into a room filled by firemen and police. The senior policeman welcomed me and asked me what I was going to do. Observing my age, he helpfully asked me if I'd done this before. I said no and clearly had no idea what to do. I told him I'd seen a film (I couldn't remember which one) in which the doctor passes a cup of tea out the window to the patient and she comes back in. OK Doc, the policeman said and shouted for a cup of tea from one of his men.

They put me in a harness. I tried to explain that in the film the doctor didn't actually go onto the ledge, but I found myself sitting beside my new patient giving her a cup of tea way above Whitehall. Amazingly it all worked and after a little chat she agreed to come back into the room to finish her tea. We firmly shut the window. The publican kindly had brought up three brandies – one for me, one for the patient and one for himself. I felt we all deserved them.

Within minutes everybody left. The traffic resumed noisily in Whitehall, and everything returned to a normal Sunday in central London. Nothing remained of the drama. I was left drinking brandy with the landlady and her husband. She was seriously depressed and willing to go into a mental health unit. So, I spent the next three hours trying to get her admitted as an emergency. I nearly succeeded with a big hospital in North London near Watford. But ten minutes later the hospital called back to say that as the pub was on the South side of Whitehall I had to start again with a hospital in Banstead. By this time my driver was incandescent – he had ten calls waiting – a chest pain in Morden, a stroke in Greenwich and a child with a severe headache in Tooting and numerous sore throats and coughs.

I couldn't leave my patient like this – she was a very nice lady. So, I dialed 999 for an ambulance. The cheerful crew arrived within five minutes and took her and her husband to the Middlesex Hospital emergency department where I had been a student. They will just have to go through all the same phone calls I thought with a slight pang of guilt.

The point of this story is that when you are first diagnosed with cancer you may well find yourself the centre of attention. Lots of professionals will talk to you offering advice. Consultants from different specialties, their registrars, nurse specialists, dieticians, physiotherapists and social workers may all visit you. But then suddenly you're on your own. Don't feel let down – just think of my Whitehall experience.

After a year as a young doctor, I knew I really wanted to do oncology, so I went to see one of the most distinguished cancer specialists of the time. Professor Gordon Hamilton-Fairley ran the research unit at the Institute of Cancer Research and then became Professor of Medical Oncology at St. Bartholomew's Hospital. He contributed a great deal to the development of chemotherapy in Britain before being tragically killed by an IRA bomb in 1975. The bomb was meant for the government minister who lived next door. Basically, I wanted to be his registrar as it would be such an excellent start in oncology. I met him in a small office next to the cancer ward at Bart's. He said that he only had ten minutes and if I impressed him there would be an application form in the post. If I didn't, I wouldn't hear from him again. He told me his registrar job was very popular and usually reserved for Bart's graduates. After a brief chat, he said I seemed like a decent enough young man and thanked me politely for coming. The next day the form was at home waiting for me.

In those days, medical interviews were far more informal. Whether I actually knew anything, or had any aptitude, for working in cancer didn't seem to worry anyone. I was likable, keen and I'd been to a good university and that was all they needed to know. I got the job.

So, I joined the cancer industry properly in 1974. Our attitude towards the disease was very different to what it is today – indeed, one of the most fascinating aspects of a career as a cancer specialist has been observing how our relationship with the condition has evolved over the years.

When I started out, we were fighting a battle against cancer – and we were going to win it as well. The papers would write constantly of 'miracle cures' for cancer. We were going to find a pill for it one day – it was just a matter of time. But miracle breakthroughs are the stuff of media and not reality.

Of course, those were different times. After all, in 1970 we had just been through a half century of extraordinary medical innovation. From the discovery of penicillin to the development of a range of vaccines, mankind had made more progress in the space of fifty years against a whole range of deadly conditions than it had in the previous couple of thousand years – and perhaps more than it will in the next couple of thousand as well. Even very poor countries had gained tremendously from our new knowledge. Antibiotics had turned once fatal diseases into little more than minor irritants, and vaccines had come close to ridding the world completely of conditions such as polio – an epidemic of which would once terrorise whole communities.

Smallpox was officially declared eradicated in 1979 by the World Health Organisation but was nearly gone except in Africa by 1970. New 'wonder pills' had revolutionised areas as diverse as birth control, depression, hypertension and stomach ulcers.

A pill for cancer? Why not? In those days new pills for just about everything were rolling out of the pharmaceutical companies' labs all the time. There was no reason why we shouldn't create a tablet for it in the same way we did for everything else. This was a challenge I firmly believed we could overcome – and I really wanted to be part of it.

Over the next thirty years, my attitude slowly changed – and so did the way we look at cancer. Language reflects the way we think about issues, sometimes deliberately, but more often unconsciously. So when I started out in my career, we always used military metaphors. What we were fighting was a battle against cancer. We waged campaigns on the disease and opened up new fronts in the struggle. There were good cells and bad cells in the body. There were sanctuary sites where cancer cells could hide in the lining of the brain. There was collateral damage to innocent normal cells through the toxicity of our drugs and radiation. One day we believed there would be total victory, and cancer would be defeated forever. *Fighting for a world without cancer* was even contemplated as a strap line for Britain's leading cancer research charity. Precision targeting to avoid collateral damage was the key to radiotherapy. Once that day came, we would all be safe from the threat.

Maybe it was because we had all grown up in the aftermath of the Second World War, and we were living in the shadow of the Cold War and the threat of the nuclear bomb. Battles were all around us, so we tended to think in those terms. But it also reflected the state of medical science at time. We had largely beaten diseases like polio, diphtheria and tuberculosis. Most bacteria were no longer a threat, and even more mysterious conditions such as depression or schizophrenia seemed to be well on the way to be overcome. We were landing men on the moon and creating the first personal computers. There seemed to be very little that technology couldn't achieve if given time and money. Everything was possible.

After the success of the lunar landing initiated by a previous President

J. F. Kennedy, the then President of the US. Richard Nixon declared his war on cancer in 1973 – often called by the media the moon-shot for cancer. The concept was beguiling – if you threw enough resources at a problem, you could do anything – land a man on the moon or even cure this terrible disease. Everything was suddenly possible. This led to the biggest expansion of biomedical research in history. Every scientist's grant application had cancer in it somewhere in those days.

Over the last three decades, the language and the attitude have both subtly changed. You didn't notice it at first. Like the transition of the leaves from summer to autumn, the steps are so gradual you are scarcely aware of them, then one day you notice the chill in the air. Something similar happened to cancer treatment. To stick with the military metaphors, we moved from a Cold War mentality to détente. This was no-longer about waging all-out war on the disease. Instead, we used words such as coping, treating, or containing using gentle treatments. The goal was to turn cancer into a chronic, controllable illness just like diabetes or hypertension. It was a disease you could live with and not die from.

The language reflected the realities. As it turned out, we never did find a cure for cancer in the sense that I along with many other young doctors thought we would in the early 1970s. It is never going to be the case that you pop along to your general practitioner, who tells you cheerfully: 'Seems like you have cancer. But never mind. Take two of these pills three times a day for a fortnight, try not to overdo things, and we'll take another look at you on Tuesday week. You should be right as rain by then." That just isn't how it is going to work, and now it doesn't look as if it ever will be.

But in another sense, we have begun to cure cancer – just not quite in the sense that we once thought we would. I don't mean to belittle the disease or to trivialize it. I've spent far too much time with cancer patients and their distraught families to ever do that. What I mean is that most cancers are treatable.

Of course, cancer can still be fatal. It often is, particularly if it is not detected early enough. But many cancers are no longer life-threatening in the way they once were. Instead, the disease has slowly morphed from a fatal into a chronic condition. Through surgery, radiotherapy, and drugs, many if not most cancers can be successfully treated.

Very often, however, the cancer will not go away – at least not a hundred percent. Instead, it will become an ongoing condition, something that needs to be constantly monitored, and occasionally treated. But – and this is the important part – it need not be something that prevents you from leading a normal, fulfilling life. I've had patients that have lived with widespread cancer for over twenty years.

It has become a manageable disease – similar to diabetes, perhaps, or to arthritis. That is true now and is getting truer with every year that passes. For example, in the US the National Institutes of Health predict that by 2030 there will be 20 million survivors of cancer in the US, a 35% increase on the 2010 total.

That is the sense in which I mean that we have, after all, 'won' the war on cancer – just not in the way we thought we would. We have learned how to live with it, and how to contain it, and how to make sure it need not stop us living life to the full. And we are still – as we shall see in the final chapter of this short book – making constant progress, which will allow patients to live even longer.

It is a huge change. But it is also one which many patients, and the healthcare systems, have not caught up with yet. I have said something about my own career and about the way cancer treatment has changed for a reason.

You've got cancer – or someone close to you has. That is the reason you are reading this book: I certainly don't imagine anyone has bought it just for light holiday reading.

You might well be thinking that your life is over. That is far from true. It is simply that you need to take control. And start organising your own care.

Back in the 1960s, when my father died, the doctors didn't tell us what was going on. That may have been wrong – it certainly seems strange from today's perspective – but even if they had done it would not have made very much difference. There was very little they could have done for him anyway. Who knows, maybe they were right to spare us the bad news for as long as possible. The range of treatments was so limited in the mid-1960s, it might well have simply upset is even more.

Now that has all changed. The two important points are these.

Your cancer will not – we hope – be fatal. But it may well be chronic, in the sense that you will probably live with it for the rest of your life. And there is far more information available – and your doctor will be far more willing to share it with you, but you need to do some work to ensure you can understand the options available.

That battle against cancer can be won. Your physician and the health care system will help you. But you must know how the system works and how to turn it to your advantage. And how to do this is precisely what the rest of this book will show you. The appendix at the end will offer you detailed guidance on using the internet as an invaluable resource.

Chapter Two: What's your life worth?

Be aware of rationing and the rapidly rising costs of the best possible care for cancer

What's your life worth? It might seem like a stupid question. Your life is worth whatever needs to be spent to keep you alive. If you were being held to ransom by a kidnapper, you would in the last resort give them everything you owned to let you live. After all, you can't take it with you. There is no point in trying to economize if you end up dead.

That surely is true of medical treatment as well. Cost doesn't matter. What counts is keeping you alive. The trouble is that is your answer. Your life is worth whatever it takes to you. But it is not necessarily true for the healthcare system as a whole.

In the last chapter, we looked at how cancer treatment has changed in the last three decades – and how it has moved from being a fatal to a chronic condition. There was one important point we haven't mentioned yet. Chronic diseases are very, very expensive to treat.

If we had won the war on cancer by developing a few simple medicines it would have been much simpler. Antibiotics, for example, cost very little to make, and not much to administer and yet have contributed to a vast improvement in healthcare. But that wasn't the way the cancer technology worked out. Instead, we have created a range of treatments, which for many people will mean the disease can be effectively contained, but which are going to cost vast sums of money over many, many years.

A few figures illustrate the point. In the UK for example, according to a report by BUPA (the largest UK private health insurer) the typical cancer patient now costs £50,000 to treat. By 2030, it's likely to have risen to £80,000. Where does all the money go? Just over a quarter of the current expenditure goes on hospital inpatient costs, not including the actual surgery – that is, simply the cost of caring for a person in hospital. Almost a quarter – 22% – goes on the cost of surgery, and 18% on drug treatments. The remainder of the budget goes on outpatient costs including diagnostic procedures, radiotherapy, cancer screening, specialist services, such as palliative care, and other community services including general practice care. It is a huge sum of money.

In the United States, as you might expect, the figures are even larger. In 2022, according to National Institutes of Health figures, to give optimal care for a brain cancer cost $125,000 for a patient over 65 in the initial phase, with an ongoing annual expenditure of nearly $15,000. Pancreatic cancer will cost $140,000 in the first year, and an ongoing expenditure of $20,000. Not all cancers are quite so expensive – in the US, for example, prostate cancer can be treated for less than $50,000. Not every medical system is quite as lavish as the American one, nor does it need to be. But none of this treatment comes cheap.

And in the US, just as in the UK, it is getting more expensive all the time. In 2020, the US spent $209 billion year on cancer treatment – that is more than the entire GDP of New Zealand. That doesn't include the financial costs to patients and their carers.

The diagnostic tests, scans, drugs and radiation therapies needed to contain complex cancer are rising in quality and effectiveness all the time – but unfortunately so is their price as well. Overall medical inflation is running at about 10% per year in nearly all countries. For optimal cancer care it's nearly 15%.

Why are cancer drugs so expensive? The truth is, these kinds of medicines are very expensive to develop, and the market for them is relatively small – they are targeting very precise forms of cancer from which fortunately only a relatively tiny group of people suffer from every year. The companies making the drugs can only turn a profit on it by charging huge sums per patient. The result is that costs are constantly rising – and are going to carry on rising all the time. And of course, many drugs in research and development never make it. The costs of developing a failed drug can be up to $1 billion. So those drugs that do make it to the market have to include these costs somehow. Shareholders want to make a profit at the end of the day. That's capitalism for you I'm afraid.

There is no point in shying away from the fact; your treatment could cost someone an awful lot of money.

It doesn't matter what kind of health care system you are in. There are going to be financial constraints on your care. In Britain, we are used to the National Health Service, paid for entirely out of taxation, always being a cash-strapped organisation. We don't expect to be getting a Rolls-Royce service. But it doesn't matter whether you are in a private system, such as in the United States, a mixed public-private system, like the ones in much of continental Europe, or with a private healthcare provider using a gold-plated medical insurance policy.

The blunt truth is this. The healthcare system wants you to live. But it is not prepared to pay any price to keep you alive. If it did, it would quickly bankrupt itself. Once you get cancer whoever is footing the bill wants to keep the cost of treating you as low as possible. You are, as the US insurers brashly put it, a 'medical loss'.

As I said earlier, the system is not there to look after you personally. It is there to look after society in general, and to provide the best possible level of care for society as a whole, and at a containable cost. Even within very well-funded healthcare systems in very rich countries, that is still true – costs have to be kept under control.

So, there is a conflict.

You want to get the best possible treatment for your cancer – after all, you only get one life.

But the system is constantly making choices based mainly on cost.

It is important that you are aware of this right at the start. The system won't own up to it. Politicians in charge of government-funded healthcare will never admit they are rationing care: there are few better ways to lose an election. And private insurers won't admit to it either. The advertising campaigns and glossy brochures are all dedicated to convincing you that no expense will be spared to provide you with the best treatment possible. Smiling attractive nurses with shiny white teeth, high tech equipment and personalised care are all emphasised in trying to win your business. But it is only partly true. They have to make a profit, just like any other business. And they can only do that by keeping costs under control.

As a patient, how can you navigate your way through this?

The first, and perhaps most important point, is to make sure you are aware of the issue of cost. If you just assume that the system will give you the best care it can simply because you need it, then you are already at a disadvantage. Remember, the best healthcare available in the world will be provided to you so long as you know your way around the system. That is true even of a relatively poorly funded and highly rationed system like Britain's NHS. But it is also true of lavishly funded private systems. They are all longer on promises than they are on actual delivery. And they all ration healthcare even if they don't admit it – and the more expensive your needs, the more they ration it.

Secondly, once you are aware of the issue, get a rough idea of the costs of your cancer care. You don't need to know it to the last hundred pounds, but you need to know how many tens of thousands are involved. The US National Institutes of Health calculations give a good rough and ready guide to the challenges you face. Brain cancer can be one of the most expensive to treat, followed by pancreatic and ovarian cancer. At the other end of the spectrum, a simple melanoma can be treated for not very much money at all. But prostate and breast cancers are becoming particularly costly to bring under control.

It is important that you get a sense early in the process of how much your illness is going to cost to treat. If it is relatively inexpensive, cost will not be any great obstacle. If you have a very expensive type of cancer, you are going to have to prepare to work a lot harder to make sure that wherever the system is looking to save money it is not going to be your life that gets sacrificed.

So, let's talk about rationing. All healthcare systems do it, but nobody talks about it. It's like using a swear word in Britain's NHS. Mention it on a hospital committee and everybody starts looking at their pens and averts their eyes from you.

Chapter Three: Rationing

What nobody tells you

Rationing is everywhere in all healthcare systems. It's a great way to reduce demand and keep costs down. You can't avoid it whether you have a gold-plated private health insurance policy or are at the mercy of your local NHS hospital. But you can understand how the system works and how to manipulate it to your advantage. Here are the five Ds of rationing explained.

- Denial
- Delay
- Deflection
- Discrimination
- Determination by committee

Denial is the most straightforward. You ask in the clinic about a new treatment you've just read about in a Sunday newspaper for your cancer, and you're told it doesn't exist. You persist and then get told it's not suitable for your cancer. Or that you don't meet the stringent criteria necessary. US medical insurance companies issue formal 'denial letters' frequently. Americans are used to arguing their case quite aggressively and frequently get them overturned. In Britain we're more constrained but all over the world those that make themselves well informed are more likely to get what they want. Information is power. In the US drug companies even post on their website's suitable responses to a denial letter about their product from an insurer.

Everybody is playing a game and you must realise it. Because for you the game could be deadly. Before making a fuss, you must be sure the treatment you want is not being denied you for a good reason. Information is the key.

Delay is a very effective form of rationing. Just imagine you have a dreadful sore throat and a temperature. You phone up your GP surgery but give up as there's no answer after ten minutes. The next day your throat feels like it's been invaded by tiny worms with sandpaper legs and is much worse. You try again. After an hour a grumpy receptionist answers. You are told the doctor is very busy and there are no appointments for two weeks. She suggests you go to a local pharmacy. But you can't get antibiotics without a prescription, so you suffer in silence for another week. You call NHS 111, the telephone advice line. After waiting for over 40 minutes, you are asked interminable questions and told to make an appointment with your GP. Then things slowly get better. So, delay is an excellent way to ration GP appointments as you are now better and don't need one. Repeat that for thousands of patients across the country and GPs can take a couple of days off to play golf every week.

Delay reduces demand very effectively. Whether it's for a diagnostic scan, an expensive blood test or even a hip replacement, delay means that some will go elsewhere maybe paying for it privately, some will die waiting and some will just forget about it. It seems cruel and unfair, but you must understand the system is not working just for your benefit whatever the snazzy straplines usually involving the word 'caring', say under the hospital's logo.

Deflection is a way of passing the buck effectively. It's widely used in our NHS to ration care. Your told that to get a booking for a particular scan you need to get a form filled by a GP or another hospital department. The responsibility has been deflected and now you suddenly become the owner of the problem. The system hopes that a sizeable number of patients will just give up so reducing demand. Even more complex deflection strategies can involve you running round in circles with several health and social agencies. You can easily get into a Catch 22 situation for which you can't extricate yourself.

Discrimination is used all the time by healthcare providers to say no. Only certain groups can access a certain service. This can be based on age, sex or even post code. The criteria can be made so incredibly complex that even the professionals don't understand the criteria being used.

Determination by committee is the fifth and most powerful rationing technique. It is perhaps the most powerful strategy. To get a certain investigation or drug treatment that may be expensive your case has to be considered by a committee of supposed experts with far more knowledge than you. This of course means a delay whilst your data is processed in advance of a meeting. You are not able to attend as you couldn't possibly understand the high-level discussion that takes place. Such committees have impressive names: multidisciplinary team, tumour board, national proton panel, resource allocation board, drugs committee. The professionals looking after you will hide behind the committee decisions and tell you that their hands are tied and no you have no right of appeal.

In Britain the ultimate rationing committee is NICE – the National Institute of Clinical Excellence. It evaluates all sorts of new diagnostics and treatments. This includes surgery, radiotherapy, and drugs. It was founded in 1999 and has been an international leader for health technology assessment. Its website proudly declares:

"NICE balances the best care with value for money across the NHS and social care, to deliver for both individuals and society as a whole.

We do this by:

- *providing rigorous, independent assessment of complex evidence to produce guidance and advice for health and social care practitioners*
- *developing recommendations that drive innovation into the hands of health and care professionals*
- *encouraging the uptake of best practice to improve outcomes for everyone".*

So, you can see immediately this is not about you at all. The methodology it uses is complex as it covers such a wide range of interventions. It tries to come to a common endpoint in its evaluation. To do this it uses the cost of single quality adjusted life year – a QALY. The official definition is as follows:

"A measure of the state of health of a person or group in which the benefits, in terms of length of life, are adjusted to reflect the quality of life. One quality-adjusted life year (QALY) is equal to one year of life in perfect health. QALYs are calculated by estimating the years of life remaining for a patient following a particular treatment or intervention and weighting each year with a quality-of-life score (on a 0 to 1 scale). It is often measured in terms of the person's ability to carry out the activities of daily life, and freedom from pain and mental disturbance".

There is still a lot of subjectivity in these assessments simply because of the wide range of treatments. How do you compare a smoking cessation clinic with high-cost drugs for lung cancer for example. Even more difficult would be a children's glue ear clinic with a hospice providing end of life care or a drop-in mental health centre. And should QALYs be age adjusted in that there's much less benefit prolonging the life of a 89 year old compared to a 40 year old? After all the normal life expectancy of the 89-year-old is a lot less. The NHS resolutely avoids any hint of ageism in its official policy, but doctors do it all the time. Again, mention that at a committee and it's as though you'd just uttered a nasty swear word.

As always, such assessments are easy to criticize but difficult to improve. NICE does spend a lot of time and effort trying to smooth over problems in its calculations. I certainly can't come up with anything better.

When you use the cost per QALY system to guide how to prioritise an always limited budget there are always going to be surprises. The smoking cessation clinic to prevent lung cancer always comes out at the lowest cost per QALY in any cancer intervention. Although not written in tablets of stone, anything costing above £30,000 per QALY will be turned down. This has not increased for 20 years which is odd as everything else costs more now. To make things even more opaque, deals are made with the big pharma companies and the NHS to reduce the price of the drug. But the details are kept secret by both NICE and the companies. And you can't get the real price by doing a Freedom of Information request. All numbers will be redacted as they are said to be commercially sensitive. I've never understood why this is necessary, but I don't write the rules.

Now you know about rationing you are empowered to work out how best to circumvent it. It all requires making sure you fully understand what you want and to be sure that it's a reasonable request. Again, information is power. But how do you get it effectively?

The results of all your tests – scans, X-rays, blood tests and biopsies are recorded in your notes in paper form and often electronically. Just ask for the key results and you should be given a printed copy. Those directly involved in your care – doctors and nurses are the first port for information. Some are more forthcoming than others. Older and more senior doctors sometimes take the attitude that its none of your business as you couldn't possibly understand all the jargon. Sometimes the most informative staff will be young and very open to sharing stuff about you. If you don't feel you're getting anywhere on no account lose your temper. Remain charming – polite and smiley but simply explain you want to understand as much as possible about your illness so you can help contribute to the healing process.

One of the problems in the NHS is time. In a busy clinic oncology doctors may be seeing up to 30 patients in a morning. New patients may be allocated 20 minutes and follow up patients 10 minutes. In private clinics here and in the US new cancer patients get an hour and a follow-up gets 30 minutes. Much more time to explain things.

So, time is rationed too. But do not despair. What you need is the correct information. The key information is the biopsy report which describes the pathology of the cancer and the imaging data showing how and where it has spread. It doesn't matter who prints it out for you – the receptionist, the clinic nurse, or the doctor. Once you have the printouts in your hand you become an empowered patient. Congratulations!

Let me give you two stories that explain how people get information about cancer. The first was a very wealthy billionaire, a man of 52 years old that had been told by his surgeons that he had pancreatic cancer that had spread to his liver. He was told to come and see me, and I would give him chemotherapy. The prognosis was hopeless, and his surgeon had been blunt – he wouldn't make it to Christmas.

He came along to my clinic, and I was frank with him. I said the drugs are not likely to work but we might be able to dampen the growth of the spreading cancer in the liver. But it's likely that eventually the cancer would start growing again and liver function would start declining. I was going to prescribe a standard chemotherapy regimen with three drugs. He didn't like the idea and asked me where he could get the best opinion in the world. He had read an article in the New York Times about a surgeon at Memorial Sloan Kettering Hospital in New York who was taking out deposits of cancer from the liver. I explained that this was unlikely to benefit him because although we could see several round holes in the liver caused by the cancer on the scans, there were almost certainly more lesions present that we could not see so there could be no complete removal and therefore no cure.

Nevertheless, he went over to New York, first class, on the next plane and directly to Memorial Hospital in Manhattan. I had given him a full medical report with packages of his biopsies and images from his scans.

He returned two weeks later saying – okay give me the chemotherapy. I asked him what happened he said it cost me $200,000 to repeat the scans and biopsy and they told me exactly what you said. He was very happy he made the journey and was now content for me to treat him with chemotherapy. For him the amount of money he'd spent was trivial but the psychological value of his American odyssey enormous.

My second story is about the power of international information transfer. I organised a course twice a year at Hammersmith Hospital for the Royal College of Radiologists called Advanced Oncology. I invited Umberto Veronesi, who was probably the world's most famous breast surgeon at the time. He was the head of the National Cancer Institute in Milan. Surprisingly he agreed to come. I was staggered and so I made a big deal out of his lecture. I billed it for noon and invited all the great and the good of breast cancer in the UK for lunch.

Ten minutes before the lecture I became very worried this was going to be a no show. Suddenly, an attractive young lady came in dressed elegantly in a leather miniskirt carrying a carousel of slides. I was very disappointed when she told me she was his registrar and I assumed she was to be a substitute. But no, she was there to load and check the slides. The great man was on his way. Indeed, at one minute before noon the door at the back of the packed lecture theatre opened and in walked in Umberto with another attractive lady. I was so relieved to see him. He gave an excellent lecture and as you can imagine everyone was thrilled that we managed to get him to come to London for our course.

The international transfer of medical information is now so commonplace that it would be impossible for knowledge of a cancer discovery in New York or Milan yesterday not to be in London today. But Italians will always have such style!

So, I can hear you saying, I don't have the bread to go to New York tomorrow and I can't speak Italian. How can I possibly be a fully informed patient? The answer of course is to be like a sponge – just soak up information from all possible sources.

Start with your doctors and nurses. Make sure you get the full details of your illness. Get the exact type of cancer confirmed – and above all get hold of a copy of the biopsy report. A biopsy is just a sample of your tissue taken from an area of your body suspected of being a cancer. Often called the histology or histopathology report, it holds the key to your diagnosis. Don't be put off by professionals telling you that you couldn't possibly understand it, after all it's your body. Obviously, you will know the likely primary site of the cancer – breast or lung for example – but the report will contain a lot more relevant information. You need it.

You also need to understand exactly where your cancer is and where it has spread to. This is determined by imaging – X-rays, scans and ultrasound. Having all this detail allows you to take control and ask the right questions about your options. I'll explain how to use all this later.

The most powerful information ally you have is the internet. But there are over a billion sites with the word cancer in them. You can't possibly look at them all. But before you can start you need the biopsy and imaging reports. Then you can seriously begin to take control.

Getting a second opinion

You will have heard of patients who get a second opinion. This is not so easy as it sounds. When I first started in oncology in the good old days of the NHS, you would just pop along to your GP, and he would fix it up for you. It was a rare event though. Your first problem with this route is the difficulty in getting a face-to-face appointment with your doctor. The second is that he won't know you from Adam and certainly know nothing about your cancer predicament. The last and most insurmountable problem is within the NHS, GP referrals are controlled and monitored by committee. That of course is being polite – what is really happening is rationing to keep the costs down. So, the chances of getting an effective second opinion through the NHS before you start treatment are now really negligble. The capacity just isn't in the system to provide this sort of service.

So, what can you do? The only way is to get a private appointment. This will cost between £250 and £350. It may be worth doing just to give you and your family peace of mind. You could persuade someone to give it you as an early birthday present.

The first problem is making sure you've got all your clinical data – imaging and biopsy reports together with the proposed treatment plan. You're quite entitled to all this information but there are still jobsworths in the NHS that delight in saying no. But it's your body and your data about you. Be polite and persistent with the consultant's secretary or the receptionist – if necessary, enlist the help of the local PALS (Patient Advice and Liaison Service) service found in every hospital. The staff are usually very nice ladies who will do their very best to get things done. If no joy just write to the consultant. On no account be rude or aggressive to anyone as doors will shut firmly in your face.

The second problem is who to see. There's no point asking the consultant that's going to treat you as they are most likely to refer you to one of their chums. Going to one of the big cancer hospitals such as Memorial in New York or MD Anderson in Houston in the US is prohibitively expensive and will set you back £100,000 or so plus the travel and hotel costs. And frankly as I explained before news travels fast in oncology so there's no real need to leave your home country.

It's vital you see someone who specializes in your type of cancer and is bang up to date. Not too young and not too old like me. The ideal age is 45 to 60 years. It doesn't matter whether they are a man or woman or what their ethnic background is. They should be taking part in clinical trials, have some sort of research activity and work in a large cancer centre. They should be publishing in the academic literature and be on the international lecture circuit.

Most such consultants do some private work. Doctors are not allowed to advertise their services directly but if you look on the websites of large private hospitals and clinics you will find them. Try these websites by searching for your type of cancer. The other way is to ask around, but I can't stress enough how important it is that they specialise in your type of cancer.

The London Clinic in Marylebone has a large oncology Department. There are about 40 oncologists who work there nearly all part time. The cancer centre is relatively new and swanky and was opened by the Queen a decade ago. It's not a bad place to start your search. I have never worked there myself but have given second opinions on patients in the hospital. It is well equipped but expensive.

www.thelondonclinic.co.uk
Another useful site is that of the Leaders in Oncology Care (LOC) in Harley St. This was taken over by Hospital Corporation of America (HCA) a decade ago and is associated with their Harley Street Clinic next door. I was HCA's adviser on cancer a few years back. Nearly all the oncologists at the London teaching hospitals go there so there are plenty of opinions to be had.

https://www.hcahealthcare.co.uk/facilities/loc-leaders-in-oncology-care
A third organization that may be useful is Top Doctors. Don't be fooled by the name – anybody can be a Top Doctor and many that are at the peak of their profession have not joined. It works like a go-compare site and the organization gets a small fee from every consultation coming from its website.

www.topdoctors.co.uk
Because I've worked mainly in London, I know the scene well. But there

are many very competent oncologists all over the UK. You can check out the websites of the local private hospitals such as Spire, Ramsay and BMI. Or you can go to Genesis Care which runs a network of fourteen private cancer clinics. I set up the first ten before they bought us out.

Once you've identified who you think could give a good opinion check out their publications over the last five years on Google Scholar. Put in their full name and see how productive they have been in areas associated with your type of cancer.

You then need to choose and book an appointment. Make sure they have as much clinical information sent to them in advance of your appointment. Take along your partner or a close friend and if you like ask if they mind you recording their recommendation on your phone. Good doctors won't mind. Taking a video is a little intrusive – I've never refused but feel a little uncomfortable. Make sure you get a copy of the report.

One trick. Some older doctors may not see you without a referral letter. But this may be difficult to obtain. As long as you have all the stuff, I've listed you'll be fine. Get an appointment and say you'll sort out the letter. You can ask your GP just for the letter or you can ask the consultant who first saw you. If you've got the info on yourself then the letter is not important. The whole charade is just a throwback to a different age of medicine when the system held all the cards, and you were just an ignorant nuisance. Times have changed!

I first got involved in a second opinion when I was a houseman (now called Foundation doctor) at the Middlesex Hospital. We had a VIP on my ward and the consultant arranged for him to have a second opinion. This was from Britain's most eminent oncologist at the time, Sir Ronald Bodley Scott who was the senior physician at Barts. It was arranged for 10:00am on a Saturday morning and I was on call for the weekend. My boss was away in Italy, so I was asked to meet and greet him in the private wing. I was called when he drew up in a chauffeur driven Rolls Royce. It was like a scene from the film 'Doctor in the House'. We went to the ward together and I introduced him to the patient. He just grunted at me. I presented the history, and he examined the patient. I arranged for coffee in the Sister's office. He asked me what sort of name Sikora was. He certainly hadn't done a current NHS diversity course. I politely said it was Polish and he asked me if I was clever. I told him I got a double first at Cambridge. That doesn't mean much he said.

He wanted me to give our patient an experimental treatment that had been pioneered in America. He said we can do it here, but you must follow my recipe to the letter. He prescribed a high dose of a drug called methotrexate. The dose would be lethal unless the antidote, folinic acid, was given 24 hours later. He wished me good luck but didn't leave me his phone number. There were no mobiles in those days anyway.

I got the methotrexate from pharmacy infused it as planned. All was well until midday on the Sunday. I'd written up for the folinic acid rescue – the antidote – after his visit. At noon I asked the ward sister where was it? She told me the pharmacy didn't have it, but it would come tomorrow. I panicked as I knew he needed to be given the antidote that day or his bone marrow would be wiped out.

Sir Ronald hadn't left me a phone number and was ex-directory. My boss was sunning himself on the Italian seaside. I then phoned the duty registrar in oncology at Barts. He jokingly said 'I see we've let old Bodley out and about again. He does this all the time. Don't worry just be by the front door of the hospital in ten minutes and you will have your drug.' I stood at the front of the hospital wondering how this was going to work. Suddenly a police car zoomed round the corner with sirens blaring and a jolly policeman gave me a box with the drug. Just amazing. The patient got it at precisely noon that day.

I hope your second opinion follows a smoother course.

Chapter Four: What is cancer anyway?

Information is power – understanding the problem is the key to finding a solution

Cancer is extremely common. One in three of us will develop the disease. By the year 2020, this number will be one in two in Europe, North America and parts of Asia. We read about it daily in newspapers and magazines and it seems to be gathering momentum. In the past, cancer and death have been strongly associated, making cancer almost a taboo topic. But this is a myth. Most people that get cancer, particularly if it is diagnosed early, will make a complete recovery. The death rate for many chronic medical conditions such as heart disease and stroke is far greater than that for cancer.

Moreover, in the last 30 years there have been dramatic strides in our understanding of what cancer is and how best to treat it. Cancers that were almost universally fatal in the past, such as Hodgkin's lymphoma and testicular cancer, are nearly completely curable now even if they have spread widely in the body. There have been tremendous improvements in the care of all cancer patients, from making the diagnosis with greater precision to following what is happening during treatment and controlling any unpleasant symptoms. We have much better information about the numbers and sort of people it is likely to affect. It is true that the disease is becoming more common. This is not because of changes in our environment as many like to believe, it's just that we live longer as a population and as cancer occurs more commonly in the elderly, so the incidence is bound to go up.

We've also managed to break through some of the taboos that used to surround the disease so that diagnosis is quite open between doctor and patient and between family and friends. But this new openness means that the need for information has never been greater. Consumerism has hit healthcare in a big way. The way health services around the world are adapting to dealing with the spiraling costs of high technology shows that no society has the perfect answer. If consumerism is used correctly, it can change the way we live and the quality of our healthcare for the better. But to avoid tilting at windmills, it must be based on fact. To have the best chance of beating cancer, you must have at least a minimal knowledge about the biology of the disease. This section will give you just that. You need to understand better what the problem is and why it is a challenging disease to treat if you're going to get the best care possible.

The cell

To understand what cancer is, we must look at how the body is made. We are all built of cells so tiny that they are only visible by a powerful microscope. About a thousand billion are needed to make a person. The cells of different tissues are specialized to have different functions. A muscle cell, for example, has tiny molecular ropes to allow it to contract. A skin cell has a tough waterproof coat to protect it from the environment. And a liver cell is a little chemical refinery continuously cleansing the blood of potential poisons. In most people these different cells work in perfect harmony, but sometimes things go wrong.

If a single cell dies, one of its many identical partners simply takes over its job. If we cut ourselves then a whole series of repair processes are brought into action. Cells start to divide, and they readily replace damaged tissue. Normal cells are dying all the time in our bodies, to be replaced by new and healthy ones. But if a cell starts to grow and divide in an abnormal way, so getting out of control, then problems can arise. Sometimes this leads to cancer, a disease of abnormal growth. To understand the basic problem, we have to look first at how normal cells grow and reproduce.

Normal cells

Normal cells consist of a membrane, cytoplasm, and nucleus. The membrane is a complex structure, which includes many protein molecules stretching across it. These project an outside piece, which acts as a receptor and an internal portion. Signals received from the outside world are transmitted through the membrane to tell the cell what to do. When we are suddenly frightened, for example, adrenaline is released into the blood stream. The cell receptors pick this up and prepare our muscles and nervous system to deal rapidly with the situation. Cell surface markers also enable the body's immune system to recognise foreign molecules of infected cells; processes that are vital in resisting and overcoming infection. In addition, the cell membrane provides a skeleton for the cell and helps maintain the correct balance of chemical inside.

The cytoplasm is a biological soup inside the cell, which contains structures vital for the working and growth of the cell. These are essential for the division into two daughter cells during growth and to produce substances by the cell as part of its everyday function.

The control plant of the cell is its nucleus. This contains material known as DNA, deoxyribonucleic acid, a chemical sequence in which information is stored and passed on from one cell to the next and indeed from one generation to the next. It is this information that determines whether, for example, a cell will be part of muscle or skin. It is also through the DNA that physical characteristics – height, hair colour, eye colour, intelligence and so on – are passed from parents to children.

All complex organisms including humans grow from a single cell by a series of events in which a cell splits into two, a process known as mitosis. During this the DNA in the nucleus of the single cell replicates itself to form two nuclei. At the same time, the cytoplasm divides that surrounds the two nuclei resulting in two cells enclosed each by a membrane. The two new cells, the daughters of the original, then divide to form four cells and so on. Sometimes the molecular machinery that controls the growth process can go wrong. Often, it's due to a change in the information carried by the DNA. This results in the formation of an abnormal cell. Many abnormal cells just die out. Some have changes that make them more able to grow rapidly and – in sites of the body where normally a differentiated cell cannot – become a cancer.

Normal cells do not become cancerous suddenly. There is a series of events that culminate in a cell growing out of control. These events take place long before the cancer becomes a recognised problem in a patient – maybe predating the actual diagnosis by several years. We know this because sometimes, purely by chance, some of the earlier changes can be seen down a microscope. In the cells lining the small airways of the lung small areas of change can be detected by looking at new patterns emerging. These changes are much more common in heavy smokers. Similarly, in the neck of the womb cervical smears can detect a pre-malignant change that heralds the onset of cancer of the cervix, which can indeed be lethal.

What actually is a cancer?
Cancer is a mass of tissue formed because of cells growing abnormally and excessively. These cells continue to grow indefinitely and without restraint. A tumour basically means a swelling. There are two types: benign and malignant. Broadly speaking benign tumours are localized. That is, they do not spread from the part of the body in which they began. They often have a clear capsule – a rim of normal tissue, which marks the limit of the cancer. They may be detected because as they grow, they

press on other important structures in the body such as blood vessels or intestines. In the skin, they cause blemishes, which can easily be seen. A simple wart is a good example of a benign tumour. On the whole, such tumours are easily removed by surgery and do not recur. It is only in rare cases, for example if a benign tumour exists deep in a vital part of the brain, that surgery is likely to cause serious damage, and is impossible.

Malignant tumours are true cancers. They are virtually never surrounded by a capsule and often erode adjacent tissues, infiltrating other parts of the body and extending with crab-like projections in all directions. Indeed, when cancer was first described it was named after the Latin for a crab as it seemed to have claws. With a few exceptions, the unequivocal feature of all malignant tumours is their ability to spread through the blood and lymph vessels and establish themselves in other parts of the body. This process is called metastasis from the two Greek words *meta* meaning next and *stasis* meaning place. The cancer cells have quite simply changed places, spreading around the body to a site at which they can grow. When they form tumours in other sites, they can cause widespread symptoms and damage critical organs such as the lung, liver, kidneys and bone marrow.

Classifying cancer

Cancer can arise in any organ of the body. The behaviour pattern of different cancers varies enormously. There are currently more than 200 classifiable sites at which tumours can arise and many of these can be broken down into further subtypes. As we fully understand the molecular basis of the abnormalities in growth control, it is likely that we will identify many individual abnormalities that represent the cause of cancer in an individual and can be targeted by designer drugs.

Tumours are classified by the site at which they originate. For example, a patient with breast cancer that has spread through the blood stream to the liver, is said to have metastatic breast cancer, not a primary liver tumour. This often causes confusion amongst patients and families who assume that it is a liver tumour rather than a tumour actually arising from the breast. Tumours are also given a name reflecting the types of tissue structure from which they are derived. A carcinoma comes from cells lining the body cavities. Such cells are found in the lung, colon, breast and prostate and form the majority of cancers. Tumours arising from the body's structural tissues, muscle, tendon, bone and cartilage are called sarcomas. Those arising from the lymphatic system are called lymphomas and cancers of the white blood cells and bone marrow, leukaemias.

Cancer symptoms

Because there are many different types of cancer, there is no one way in which it first draws attention to itself. What happens depends on the site and size of the tumour or on any spread of the disease as well as on any other medical problems a patient may have. So, a small tumour of the throat will rapidly create an ulcer, preventing closure of the vocal cord while speaking and so leading to hoarseness. In this way a relatively tiny tumour, no more than 2mm in diameter, can produce the alarming symptom of persistent hoarseness driving the patient to a doctor rapidly and usually long before the tumour has time to spread.

Patients with lung cancer on the other hand, often show no unusual symptoms until relatively late. Most of such patients are smokers who are used to frequent coughing, shortness of breath, and even occasional chest pains, all the features of a growing lung cancer. By the time something really novel develops such as coughing up a small amount of blood, the tumour has firmly established itself. Pain comes from the pressure on or the destruction of tissues containing nerve fibre endings. The centres of most organs contain no nerve endings, and it is only when that outer lining is stretched that the patient notices that there is something seriously wrong.

Being aware of symptoms that may well be related to cancer is a vital component of health education. An organ not functioning properly is one symptom; there are many others that are much less specific. These include a feeling of tiredness, weakness, weight loss, fever, nausea and sweating at night. How these effects are produced is not always clear. The most likely explanation is that substances are released by tumour cells, which trigger the symptoms indirectly. Of course, any of these may be caused by medical problems other than cancer. The most important thing you can do to help yourself is consult your doctor immediately if you have any persistent symptoms for more than two weeks. In most cases it will almost certainly have a trivial cause and a false alarm but in some it may well be due to cancer or some other serious illness.

If you want to know more about 'what is cancer' I can strongly recommend this excellent primer by one of my old registrars Professor Nick James. It's now in its second edition and is the clearest explanation I've ever had the pleasure of reading.

Cancer: a very short introduction by Nick James 2nd edition 2023 Oxford University Press.

Chapter Five: How cancer is diagnosed

The tests, the scans and the dilemma of screening

Finding out if you have cancer

Every day in Britain a thousand patients are diagnosed as having cancer with no seasonal variation. The UK falls behind most European countries in the overall survival at 5 years – the key international metric of cancer outcomes. The reasons for this are complex but increasing evidence points to delay in the diagnostic process being the single most important factor. Data looking at one year survival shows even greater disparity from Europe. The one-year survival statistic is mainly determined by delays in diagnosis and not the quality of care for the four common cancers: breast, lung, prostate and colon. If you have symptoms, you simply need to get a move on.

So, you've noticed some problems that suggest that you may possibly have cancer. At what point do you do something about it? We call this the symptom threshold. It differs enormously between people of different ages, between men and women, between people with different levels of education and socio-economic backgrounds and ethnicity. It's like a pot that is bubbling away boiling on the stove. At some point it will spill over, and action must be taken – how long do you let it bubble up? The symptom threshold varies for the perceived importance of what's wrong. A persistent sore throat or vague abdominal bloating are far less worrying to most people than coughing or vomiting up blood. A myriad of other problems which grumble along are thought as much less serious and are slow to get over the threshold to seek medical attention.

Once you admit you need help what should you do? Here in Britain your first port of call will be your GP surgery. Everyone has a GP but over the last three years it has become far more difficult to access help by getting a face-to-face appointment. Initially, this was due to COVID but even as we recover from this, appointments with GPs are rationed and difficult to obtain. You will find yourself being fobbed off by a receptionist who tries to push you into another direction. It's just the rationing by delay and deflection I described in chapter 3. If you're offered a phone call from the doctor, take it. At least you can get an action plan started.

The main thing is to always be persistent. Be polite, do not lose your temper do not use unpleasant words or start shouting down the phone. That will do you no good whatsoever. Just be pleasant and persistent by phoning back again and again even if you must wait half an hour for the phone to be answered. One of my favourite broadcasters told me that she said to the receptionist – we can do this the easy way or the hard way. The latter involved calling back at hourly intervals. If you're really struggling to access your GP, call NHS 111. This is a free telephone help service everywhere in the UK. You can use it online but it's best to allow the operator to go down their computer algorithm. Few people appreciate that the phone handlers are not trained in medicine. After a week's induction, they stick to the rigid script of the computer and are paid around £12 an hour – just above the minimum wage.

I recently chaired the Northeast London 111 service provider for three years and was amazed how effective it was for many things. Mostly trivial coughs, colds and sneezes. Unfortunately for cancer it's not so good as you need to get hospital-based tests to get sorted. But it's certainly worth trying as there are nurses and GPs available to the call centre to provide advice. They may well call you back if any red flag symptoms from you are fed into the computer. This NHS link has a great list of things to say if you are getting the run around. Remember seat 20B and use them.

https://www.nhs.uk/conditions/cancer/symptoms/

If you get really stuck the alternative is to go to the emergency department of a big hospital. The problem with that is that emergency departments are meant for people with major injuries, heart attacks, strokes and so they're not catering for people with complex symptoms that need to be evaluated by tests and scans.

Over the last decade urgent care centres have been set up by the NHS often adjacent to the emergency department. These are the ideal places if you really can't get through to your GP. Sometimes they have a common entrance with the emergency room and sometimes they are separate but in a convenient location where you can park easily. The important thing is to use them get you started on the investigative chain as quickly as possible.

My advice whenever you seek medical help is to take a good book or a laptop and assume you're going to be waiting endlessly. If you're seen within ten minutes – fantastic, but managing your own expectations is essential to prevent frustration. Don't be rushing off to another appointment afterwards or leave your car in some expensive high rise car park around the corner or arrange to go to the theatre with a new girlfriend that evening. You could be there for a long time. The system simply doesn't value your time at all. Once you get through the initial assessment almost certainly some tests will be requested.

There are three types of tests for cancer. The first are blood tests. These are not usually very specific. They look at your general health, how your blood count is doing, how your liver and kidneys are functioning, if there's any inflammation and so on but they don't really tell you much about your cancer situation. Recently a few cancer blood tests are being trialed but they're not yet that effective. The Holy Grail of cancer testing is to have something in your GP surgery that gives you an instant read out. You leave the surgery knowing whether you have or don't have cancer. A lot of hype is made of them through public relations companies, so articles repeatedly appear in the papers. One example is the Galleri test from a Californian company called Grail. Britain's NHS has partnered with the company to study many people with no symptoms to see if it can detect cancer early. It works by examining alterations in the blood of DNA coming from any cancer cells. Within the trial the test is free, but it is on sale in the US for nearly $1,000 a test. I predict it will be dumped quietly in the next two years as it produces too many false positives. This means worrying a lot of people unnecessarily. And what are GPs supposed to do with them – send them all for total body scanning? Just not possible – we simply don't have the capacity.

The second type of test is to create an image of the relevant part of your body that is causing you problems. This could be a simple X-ray of the chest or an ultrasound which uses sound waves to look at structures inside the body. More complex and therefore more expensive are scans such as the CT (Computer Tomography) or an MRI (Magnetic Resonance Imaging). These look the detailed anatomy of the internal organization of the body. If there is a cancer this will show up provided it's large enough. All imaging systems, however fancy have size limit below which nothing can be detected. This varies in different parts of the body but most tumours below 0.5 cm in diameter will go undetected but then they rarely cause symptoms.

For certain types of cancer there are designated clinics for sorting patients out quickly. The best example is the breast clinic for people with breast lumps. Only one in ten will turn out to be cancer. The majority are benign, but everybody needs sorting out. Breast clinics were set up 30 years ago to help with the mammography screening programme. In the breast clinic there will be a surgeon, a pathologist and an oncologist who will examine you take a biopsy and an ultrasound and give you the result the same day. That was the beauty of the concept. You know when you leave the hospital that day whether you had cancer or not and what was going to be done about it. Many even have the date for their first treatment.

Round the country there is a lot of variation in access both to GPs and possible cancer referral clinics. GPs know what's available locally and refer you to where they think is most appropriate. Symptoms in different parts of the body will make get you referred to the most appropriate site within the NHS. So, chest symptoms will get you referred to a chest clinic, abdominal symptoms to gastroenterology, those of bladder or prostate disease to a urologist and so on. It's most unlikely your GP will refer you directly to an oncologist as the first entry point into secondary care as we call the general hospital system. This is simply because the first treatment for most cancers is some sort of surgery.

Sometimes getting sorted out is just painfully slow. If this is the case, you may want to consider going privately for a single consultation to beat the queue. This will cost between £200 – 300 and may well give you peace of mind. Outside the NHS you're entitled to go anywhere you like. You may want to go to a big city away from where you live. Enquire what the waiting times are for a new patient with suspected cancer from the GP's receptionist. Ask friends and family for advice.

If you are thought likely to have cancer by your GP, there is a system called the two-week wait. I was involved in the creation of this fast track in the year 2000. I was a member of our Department of Health's Expert Advisory Group on Cancer. We met every month in Whitehall, and it was chaired by the Chief Medical Officer. It seemed reasonable to prioritise those patients that GPs thought might have cancer. The two-week rule means that if a GP thinks you have cancer you the hospital service had to see you within two weeks. This didn't mean you got treated within two weeks though. All it meant is you'd be seen by someone and then there could be a wait to get the necessary investigation such as the CT scan. The whole two-week wait concept was a pragmatic way of trying to overcome the delays inherent in a severely under capacitised system.

Over the last 22 years things have not got much better. The biggest failing of the two-week wait was the observation that only 25% of cancer patients came through it. Not only that, by far the majority of patients referred didn't actually have cancer at all. Even the most experienced GPs struggle to sort out the symptoms of cancer from those of a whole host of other benign much less serious illnesses. In Europe and in North America people laughed at us for having this system. Surely, they said, everybody who's got symptoms that could be cancer gets seen within two weeks anyway! In France you'd get a scan the next day in Germany within one week and so on but here we've tolerated this second-class service for so many years. That's why our survival results in Britain are well below the European average – it's not the quality of treatment but diagnostic delays.

And of course, COVID hasn't helped recently. It has increased the delays to meet targets even in even in 2023. If you've been referred under the two-week wait and you're not seen within two weeks, you need to make a fuss. Go back to your GP and complain. Call the secretary at the hospital for the relevant clinic but remember to be charming.

The other trick used by clinics is that the two-week wait doesn't specify what will happen when you're seen in the clinic. You may be seen by junior doctor and just a simple blood count requested. You are asked to come back in a month for the result. That's going against the spirit of fast tracking. At that point you need to push you for whatever test you're on the waiting list for. If it's a scan, can you afford to get it privately quickly? In London and most cities, you will easily find CT and MRI appointments on Google for tomorrow for around £300 at most. Sure, you will need someone to sign the request form but often the imaging service will get one of their clinicians to do this. Alternatively see if you can expedite it in the NHS by politely phoning up the imaging department and saying that you'll take any appointment at any time even a short notice cancellation. Say your symptoms are getting worse. It's your life after all – so what can be more important than getting sorted out quickly at this stage.

The ultimate diagnosis of cancer can only be made by obtaining a small piece of the abnormal tissue and examining it under the microscope. That is what is meant by a biopsy. It inevitably means an invasive process to obtain tissue. It may just be a fine needle that is put into a lump to extract a few cells or a much thicker bore needle to take a bigger sample. It may involve the surgical excision of a suspect lump or a lymph node or just a painless snip of an abnormal area in your colon with tube put into the rectum. Some biopsies are carried out under with an imaging technique, such as and ultrasound or either CT or MRI scanning. This is to ensure that the right bit inside your body is sampled.

All biopsies are placed in a fixative solution and sent to the pathology laboratory. When they get there, the pathology technician slices them onto microscope slides. The slides are stained with special stains to make characteristics of the cells' architecture more visible. The pathologist looks at the tissue down the microscope and a report is written. This will give the fine details of the cancer and most importantly its grade. This tells you how much it it is deviating from the normal cells from which it arose.

It is vital that you get hold of that report. It contains the key information about you, the optimal treatment and your chances of being cured. The only exception to a biopsy being vital is with a blood cancer such as leukaemia and myeloma. Here a simple blood sample can give the diagnosis. It's really the equivalent of a biopsy.

You need to know three things from the combination of your scans and biopsy.

1. Where is the primary tumour coming from?
2. What is its exact type and grade from the biopsy?
3. How far has it spread – what is its stage?

With those three key pieces of information, you have become a fully empowered patient.

Your chances of survival are driven by the stage of the disease at presentation. For all four of the major cancers – lung, breast, colon and prostate – Stage I disease has a nearly 90% 5-year survival. This is disease confined to the primary organ in which it arose. Stage 2 disease represents extension of the cancer to neighbouring lymph nodes or surrounding tissues whilst stage 3 and 4 are increasing spread of cancer around the body. Staging systems are slightly different for cancers in different parts of the body but the principle is the same. The outcome drops precipitously as the stage increases. Any delay is likely to result in upstage migration and therefore result in poorer survival for that cancer. More advanced cancer is more expensive to treat as it may involve significantly more radiotherapy and chemotherapy and so achieving an earlier diagnosis could well be cost effective.

By 2040 a new era of sophisticated molecular diagnostics will bring far better prediction of individual cancer risk. It will enable the selection of populations for screening for DNA mutations and epigenetic changes. Unique signature sequences will be discovered and be used to identify people with early cancer at defined sites. The current pan-cancer tests (for any cancer) are not specific enough to be effective and will create profound problems for the worried well. They will be replaced shortly by a new generation of far more effective analytical tools which will gradually evolve in precision over the next decade.

The most important thing you need to know about cancer is that the earlier the diagnosis is made the better the outcome – this applies right across the world in rich and poor countries alike. So, if you do think you've got cancer, especially if you've already been seen and told that it may well be cancer you need to get a sense of urgency into your investigations.

Cancer screening

Cancer screening seems so logical to all healthcare workers and patients alike. We all know that early cancer is curable in most cases and later stage disease is not. So, picking up cancer before a patient has symptoms would seem ideal. The problem is that none of the tests available are perfect. And the resources spent on screening may well be better spent on speeding up appropriate referral of symptomatic patients. Let us consider the advantages of screening along with the downside for the common cancers.

Cancer screening is defined as the systematic application of a test to individuals who have not sought medical attention because of symptoms. It can be opportunistic (offered to patients consulting their doctor for another reason) or population-based (covering a predefined age range, with elaborate call and recall systems). Britain's NHS has rightly concentrated on the latter, allowing it to be at the global forefront of population screening procedures. The risk of dying from a cancer always increases with its degree of spread or stage.

The aim of screening is to detect cancer in its earliest, asymptomatic phase. The problem is that many screening tests are relatively crude, and cancers can have metastasized before they are detected by screening. Sensitivity varies between tests. A 100% sensitive test detects all cancers in the screened population. The most rigorous means of calculating sensitivity is to determine the proportion of expected cancers not presenting as interval cases between screens. Good cancer registration is essential when making this calculation. Specificity is the proportion of negative results produced by a test in individuals without neoplasia. A 100% specific test gives a positive result only when a cancer is present with no false positive results at all.

The problem is that none of our screening tests have 100% sensitivity and specificity. The investigation of patients without cancer is a major factor in the cost of screening. The advantages and disadvantages of screening must be considered carefully and vary between cancers and tests. The three main problems in assessing the benefit of any screening test for cancer are lead-time bias, length bias and selection bias. All impair the effectiveness of screening as a method of reducing cancer mortality.

Lead-time bias advances the diagnosis but does not prolong survival, for example when the disease has already spread but the primary tumour is still small. Individuals die at the same time as if the disease had not been detected early. Length bias results in the diagnosis of less aggressive tumours. Rapidly growing cancers with a poorer prognosis present in the screening interval, reducing the value of the screening process. Selection bias occurs even in the best-organized healthcare systems. Worried but healthy individuals (who would present early with cancer symptoms) comply with screening obsessionally, whereas less well-educated and socially disadvantaged individuals do not. In the UK, compliance with the NHS breast cancer screening programme varies between communities depending on relative deprivation, ethnicity, and degree of social exclusion.

Rational decision-making about cancer screening requires a detailed analysis of factors that can vary between populations: The cancer should be common, and its natural history properly understood. This enables a realistic prediction of the proposed test's likely value. The test should be effective (high sensitivity and specificity) and acceptable to the population. Cervical smears are difficult to perform in many Islamic countries, where women prefer not to undergo vaginal examination, and the take-up rate for colonoscopy is low in asymptomatic individuals because it is uncomfortable and sometimes unpleasant. The healthcare system must be able to cope with patients who produce positive results and require investigation. This can be a particular problem in getting started.

Ultimately, screening must improve the survival rate in a randomized controlled setting. The natural history of many cancers can change over time for reasons that are poorly understood and lead to increasing overdiagnosis in cancer screening. In Europe, the incidence of stomach cancer has decreased dramatically over recent few decades. However, breast cancer deaths reached a peak in the UK in 1989 and have decreased slightly each year since, associated with earlier stage at presentation, better care pathways with increased personalization and a significant increase in ductal carcinoma-in-situ.

Well-meaning lobby groups often exercise political pressure to implement screening programmes even when their effectiveness is undemonstrated. Manufacturers of equipment and suppliers of reagents can exercise commercial pressure. In fee for service based provider systems such as the USA, there is a huge financial inducement for doctors to screen and investigate, because doing nothing simply earns no money. The launch of the NHS breast screening service by the UK government in 1989 was viewed by many as a pre-election vote winning exercise rather than a rational public health intervention. There are now similar pressures to introduce prostate cancer screening, although uncertainty remains about the management of men with slightly elevated concentrations of prostate specific antigen (PSA).

Many groups (governments, medical charities, health-maintenance organizations, professional bodies) have produced their own cancer screening guidelines. These vary widely between countries, reflecting bias in interpretation of evidence and cultural values in the practice of medicine; for example, annual PSA testing and digital rectal examination in men >50 years of age are recommended by the American Cancer Society (ACS) but not advocated in most other countries. The USA carries out more cancer screening on populations that can afford it, through either insurance or direct payment, than any other country.

The incidence of a particular cancer in a country and the economics of screening must be considered carefully e the cost of the technology required must correspond with the gain. Low-cost, direct-inspection techniques for oral and cervical cancer by non-professional health workers seem attractive for achieving tumour downstaging and hence better survival results; however, the overall effectiveness of cervicoscopy programmes in India and China has been surprisingly poor. It remains to be seen whether staining with acetic acid can enhance specificity at little extra cost.

A major cost in instituting any screening procedure is in informing the public and then developing the logistics, often under difficult geographical conditions. Cultural barriers can be insurmountable without better education, particularly of girls, who as mothers will become responsible for family health. Low technology tests have low specificities; as a result, hard-pressed secondary care facilities are inundated with patients with nonlife-threatening abnormalities. Detailed field assessment, preferably in a randomized setting, is essential before firm recommendations can be made, but political factors often interfere with this. The well-meaning charitable donation of second-hand mammography units to some African countries has led to a haphazard introduction of breast screening in populations where the incidence of breast cancer is low and there are few resources to deal with abnormal results.

The ultimate measure of success in a screening programme is a demonstrable reduction in mortality in the screened population. However, this needs large numbers of individuals, and at least 10 years' assessment for most of the common cancers. Although randomized studies can show conclusive benefit, it must be remembered that the expertise and professional enthusiasm available to a study population can be considerably greater than that achievable under subsequent field conditions. Quality of mammography interpretation and investigation of breast abnormalities are good examples and may explain the relatively disappointing results of breast screening in practice. Case-control studies using age-matched individuals from the same population and non-randomized comparisons between areas providing and not providing screening can give useful indications but are not as conclusive as randomized trials. Surrogate measures of effectiveness can be used to assess a programme with relatively small numbers of patients soon after its implementation but are insufficient to prove that screening saves lives. When a population is first screened, a higher than expected incidence of cancer should be seen because screening is detecting cancer that would not present with symptoms for several years. Subsequent rounds of screening are less productive.

Tumour down-staging is a second measure of impact. An increase in early-stage cancer detection and, consequently, a reduction in advanced disease are expected over 3–5 years. The third, short-term evaluation is a comparison of the survival of screen-detected patients with those presenting symptomatically. Success in terms of these three indices is not necessarily translated into a useful screening programme. In the 1970s, a study of routine chest radiography and sputum cytology to detect lung cancer showed a 5-year survival of 40% in screen-detected patients, compared with an overall figure of 5%, but reduced mortality from lung cancer has not been seen in large populations. Here I will describe the current UK screening activities:

Cervical cancer
Cervical cytology reduces the incidence of and mortality from cervical cancer. Abnormalities in the sampled cells called dyskaryosis and cervical intraepithelial neoplasia are early markers of malignancy. This

identifies a group of women in whom more intense local treatment and subsequent surveillance are required. The incidence of cervical cancer was decreasing before the introduction of screening, but the rate of decrease has been significantly greater in countries with population-based screening programmes. The test is cheap, safe and usually effective, but depends on the skills of the screening cytologists who are relatively poorly paid and often demotivated, which has led to errors. Computer scanning has proved difficult to implement.

New technologies, including liquid-based cytology, thin-layer methods and human papillomavirus (HPV) DNA hybrid capture analysis, are beginning to increase specificity. Many populations with a high incidence of cervical cancer exhibit a high prevalence of certain HPV subtypes, and screening for HPV DNA by polymerase chain reaction (PCR) analysis can be valuable in identifying high-risk women. Clinical trials of HPV vaccines are underway and may further reduce the incidence of cervical cancer.

The current recommended frequency of screening by age is 25 years for the first invitation; 25–49 years 3-yearly; 50–64 years 5-yearly; 65 years only those who have not been screened since age 50 or have had recent abnormal tests.

Breast cancer
More work has been undertaken on screening for breast cancer than any other cancer. Bilateral mammography – X-rays of both breasts is now standard. Many randomized controlled studies, case-control studies and geographical area comparisons demonstrate its benefit. In the UK, the NHS Breast Screening Programme reported that 75% of women aged 50–64 years invited for screening in were tested (1.2 million individuals) and almost 7000 cancers were detected – a yield of 0.006%. A well-organized quality control process is established, and breast surgeons have been meticulous in collecting data and making them public. Quality standards have been set for various components of the programme and an annual review is produced. The NHS breast screening programme provides free breast screening every 3 years for all women aged 50 years. Because the programme is a rolling one that invites women from general practices in turn, not every woman is given an invitation as soon as she is 50 but will receive her first invitation before her 53rd birthday.

There is no doubt that the UK Breast Screening Programme saves lives, but it is difficult to assess the true cost per life saved; estimates range from £250,000 to £1.3 million. Critics want to see the money spent on ensuring the application of best practice once a diagnosis has been made. A balanced view would be to continue with screening but to ensure that systems are established to deal with all patients effectively, however they present. In developing countries, 80% of patients with breast cancer present with advanced disease. Public and professional education and effective referral networks for simple basic surgery are more effective than mammography. There is no evidence that formal teaching of regular breast self-examination has any impact on mortality. The future of mammography is to develop suitable interpretation based on artificial intelligence.

Colorectal cancer

This normally presents with symptoms of intestinal obstruction or rectal bleeding and consequent anaemia. Small tumours that have not invaded the muscle coat of the colon are easier to cure than those that have done so. In many individuals, cancer evolves from polyps, even when there is no family history; thus, identification and endoscopic removal of polyps seems reasonable. Increased yield and fewer patients presenting with advanced stage disease have been demonstrated with both faecal occult blood tests (FOBTs), immunological tests for blood and colonoscopy, but the survival benefit is less certain.

About 10% of patients with colorectal cancer have a family history of the disease and, because their relatives are at increased risk, genetic testing can form part of a more intensive screening programme. Better technology might improve specificity. Detection of abnormal DNA fragments in stool combined with virtual colonoscopy using CT scans may revolutionize the early detection of colorectal cancer without the need for endoscopy.

The NHS Bowel Cancer Screening Programme offers screening every 2 years to all men and women aged 60–69 years. People over 70 years old can request a screening kit by calling a freephone helpline. NHS Digital runs a single Bowel Cancer Screening system for England that maintains organization-related information, manages the lists of people eligible for screening, sends invitations and manages appointments, sends out test kits, records test results and provides operational and strategic reports.

The enigma of prostate cancer screening

In the USA and much of Europe, the prevalence of prostate cancer has increased by dramatically in the last 10 years. Greater longevity is partly responsible, but the principal reason is earlier detection using serum

PSA testing. Post-mortem examinations of men aged over 70 years have consistently shown that at least 50% have undetected prostate cancer. When PSA screening is introduced in asymptomatic populations, the reported incidence of the disease increases dramatically for several years. Several techniques are being developed to improve the performance of the PSA assay in distinguishing aggressive from indolent cancer. These include the use of free and complexed PSA ratios, PSA density (relating serum PSA concentration to gland volume), age-adjusted PSA, rate of increase of PSA and variation in the cut-off level.

As holistic genomic and proteomic methods become more widely used, it is likely that improved understanding of the natural history of the disease in an individual will lead to more personalized therapy after needle biopsy to access tissue. The best treatment for screen-detected patients has not been determined. Many die of another condition with no morbidity caused by their prostate disease. Localized prostate cancer can be managed by radical surgery or radiotherapy, or by doing nothing. Younger patients favour more active treatment but must cope with the potential adverse effects, which include incontinence, impotence, strictures and disordered bowel habit that often persists for many years.

A large, population-based study from the USA has shown no survival advantage after 11 years in men offered intensive screening. An authoritative review by the UK Department of Health concluded that there is currently no place for screening programmes, but that there is a need for a properly conducted randomized trial. Current UK practice is not to deny PSA testing to men over 50 years of age who request it and have been given reliable information about its benefits and hazards. Although evidence does not yet support population screening for prostate cancer, there is considerable demand for the PSA test among men worried about the disease. In response to this, the Prostate Cancer Risk Management Programme was introduced over a decade ago. This provides high-quality information to enable men to decide whether or not to have the PSA test based on available evidence about risks and benefits. After considering this information, and in discussion with their general practitioners, men aged >50 who choose to have the test can do so free of charge, on the NHS. However, PSA still remains a useful investigation in all men with symptoms of urinary outflow obstruction.

Other cancers

Various lobby groups or commercial providers often call for a screening of other cancers such as skin, ovary, endometrium, and thyroid. Although an investigation of abnormal symptoms is fully warranted, only rigorous population-based research can validate the cost-effectiveness of introducing new screening programmes. The future new technologies such as the microanalysis of circulating DNA, so-called liquid biopsy, could radically change the situation.

Future changes in cancer screening will lead to profound ethical, educational, commercial, and medical challenges. Completion of the Human Genome Project, the ability to handle large volumes of sequence data, and rapid and inexpensive assays for mutations using gene-chip technology will transform the assessment of cancer risk. Commercial pressures have caused the major pharmaceutical companies to invest heavily in genomics, and their interest will lead to the discovery of new drugs and more specific tailoring of therapies to individual patients. It is likely that groups of individuals with no family history of cancer will be identified as being at significantly increased risk of developing cancer. Devising optimal screening schedules for such groups will be a major challenge.

The biggest problem of all is motivating the customers. The compliance rate varies enormously across the world, driven by education, socioeconomic factors and deprivation. The educated worried well are likely to go for every free test offered by the health system. The socially excluded residents of the neighbouring poorer districts on the wrong side of the tracks will not visit the doctor until they have advanced stage 4 cancer. And yet private clinics offer top of the range health screening for more than £3000 of scans and tests to the gullible wealthy with no evidence of benefit. To save lives most effectively, we must target the poor. Yet we all know the problem – the system is cumbersome for everyone. Consumer organizations such as budget airlines, supermarkets and online shopping systems make it easy for everyone to navigate their offerings. In this digital age the smartphone is the way forward; yet my wife still gets 'snailmailed' for her breast screening with a poorly set out, rather unfriendly letter giving her a specific time and place to turn up. No chance to book online. Making everything convenient is the key for everybody.

And as we all know, the politics of breast cancer means that everybody gets an incomprehensible leaflet talking about risk and deliberately undermining the validity of the process. No wonder many women simply ignore the invitation. NHS population-based cancer screening is for breast, cervical and colorectal cancer only and has an excellent call-recall system. The latter comes from general practitioner lists so if the addresses are wrong in the surgery, no invitation comes. The key problems in all three programmes are the same: clunky access systems for clients, huge variations in uptake, lack of downstream processing capacity, workforce shortages at all levels, confusion in management – local, community, NHS England, Public Health England (the euphemism used is multi-layered), lack of interest in primary care and no short-term positive feedback.

Chapter Six: How cancer is treated

Getting the best treatment plan for you

Before explaining some of the treatments that are used to eradicate cancer, you need to understand the health system and how it functions once the diagnosis is made. As you now know the most likely way in which your doctors know you have cancer is from a biopsy, a small piece of tissue removed either surgically, sometimes under anaesthetic, or just by taking a needle sample from a lump. Sometimes a surgeon will operate to remove the cancer and that may be the only step required to cure it. There are many other treatments: more specialised surgery, radiotherapy, chemotherapy, hormone treatment and a whole range of specialist equipment that can be used in the battle against the disease.

The person that will normally coordinate the process is the oncologist derived from the word *onkos* in Greek meaning swelling. Oncologists come in several shapes and sizes, but all predominantly treat cancer. There are surgical oncologists who specialize in the surgery of cancer, radiation oncologists (called in some countries such as Britain clinical oncologists) who give radiotherapy, and medical oncologists that specialise in chemotherapy – giving drugs to destroy or control cancer.

In addition, there are a variety of research-based physicians that may treat only patients with a particularly rare form of cancer and nothing else. All may well have a place in your care. Usually, it will be a team effort. The whole team of different specialists usually meets regularly to discuss all the patients under their care. Such meetings are called tumour boards in North America and multi-disciplinary teams (MDT) in Europe.

Although cancer is common, many hospitals still do not have a full-time oncologist. Instead, a specialist may visit from a large cancer centre on a weekly or less regular basis to conduct a clinic and see patients. Within the hospital hierarchy, there will be a specialist responsible for your care. They are called a consultant in the UK or an attending physician in North America. Some may have an academic title from the University in which they teach such as Professor or Senior Lecturer. Under the boss will be a team of doctors including those training in the specialty and increasingly nurses who may specialize in the treatment of a single type of cancer. All can be very helpful in providing the information you need to make sure you are getting the best care possible. You need to find out who's who in your area so ask around – your GP, friends who have been patients, and any local hospital and cancer centre websites.

By the time you see a cancer specialist a diagnosis will have been made. Drawing up a plan of care is the next step. For the many curable cancers, it is vital that this plan is tailored to the individual. The best chance you have of being cured lies in getting the best possible care early on in the disease. The first thing the oncologist will do is to ask a lot of questions again and then examine you. They will then review the investigations you've had including all the imaging, pathology report of the biopsy and other tests. Once the type of cancer has been determined, the next thing is to *stage* it.

Staging just means analyzing the likely routes of spread in the body to see how far the cancer has travelled before your treatment. Clearly if treatment is to be successful, it has to eradicate every cancer cell in your body. Staging enables the treatment to be tailored more appropriately to your individual needs and gives you a better indication of what your chances of being cured are. This is called your prognosis.

There are several staging systems often adapted to the anatomy of the organ in which the cancer has arisen. The simplest is Stage I to IV using Roman numerals. Stage I cancers are confined to the primary site with no spread at all; Stage II to local lymph nodes; Stage III more widely to nodes and Stage IV to other organs around the body. The outcome or prognosis gets poorer as the stage advances.

Another commonly used staging system is called TNM. This was developed by a committee of the UICC (Union for International Cancer Control) in Geneva. In this system, the letter "T" stands for tumour; T1 implies a small tumour and T4 is a very large tumour. Other numbers and letters are added to denote different sites of the body. 'N' stands for nodes; the lymph nodes draining the organ in which the tumour is found. Enlarged lymph nodes or glands containing growing tumours are classified N1, 2 or 3 depending on the size, site and number of nodes. 'M' denotes metastases, the distance spread of the disease, which are either M1 or absent M0. So, a small cancer with a good prognosis may be T1N0M0 which will have a much better outlook that a T3N2M0 stage. The TNM concept provides a more precise analysis than the simple Roman numeral system. By knowing the stage a cancer has reached, your oncologist will have a good idea of your chance of recovery.

The second piece of information that will help in the choice of the optimal treatment plan is the *grade* of the tumour. This refers to the degree of malignancy, that is, how fast a tumour is growing or dividing. High-grade tumours are more abnormal, and the cells divide more frequently, consequently they tend to grow rapidly, invade widely and are more likely to spread to distant sites. Under the microscope they can easily be distinguished from the surrounding normal tissues. At the other end of the spectrum, low-grade tumours are relatively similar to the surrounding tissue, grow more slowly and are less likely to spread. They have relatively few cells, which are dividing. Sometimes the grade of the tumour is given as a number. Grade 1 is of low grade and so has a better outcome than grade 3. The combination of stage and grade provides the oncologist with a fair idea of what is likely to happen and can be used to decide on the best treatment possible for a particular patient as well as predicting the likely outcome.

Checklist – key questions on your treatment plan
1. What type of cancer is it?
2. How big is the primary?
3. Has it spread outside the primary tissue to anywhere else in the body?
4. Has it spread to lymph nodes?
5. What stage is the tumour?
6. What grade is the tumour?
7. What is the proposed treatment?
8. Are there other options?
9. Where will this treatment be done?
10. When will I start treatment?
11. What are the chances of the cancer being cured?
12. Can I have a copy of the biopsy and the most important imaging reports?

Surgery
Surgery is often used to remove tumours. If all the cancer cells are removed cleanly, then it may be possible to cure the cancer by surgery alone. However, depending on the size, type and location of the tumour, it may not be possible to remove all of it. If some cells are left behind, they will grow again to form another tumour or may spread to other parts of the body unless they are treated. Radiotherapy and chemotherapy are often used after surgery to try to stop the cancer coming back and spreading.

Surgery is sometimes used in the diagnosis of cancer, when a biopsy is performed to remove a small piece of tissue for testing in a laboratory.

Surgery can also be used to assess or 'stage' the cancer. As we have seen staging is a method of describing the size and spread of a tumour. A biopsy may show how advanced a tumour is depending on the characteristics of the cells, and sometimes an operation is needed to see how large a tumour has grown or if it has spread.

Reconstructive surgery can be used to reshape parts of the body that have been removed or altered during surgical treatment for cancer. Breast reconstruction after a mastectomy is a commonly used example of reconstructive surgery.

Surgery is the oldest form of treatment of cancer. The Greeks and Romans were skilled at tumour removal and sometimes cured patients with what would have been a very primitive operation. There were no anaesthetics or antiseptics. Antibiotics to prevent post-operative infection weren't dreamt of and the chances of an operation being successful were therefore minimal. Nowadays things have changed. Surgery has become a scientific discipline in which detailed knowledge of the structure and function of the body along with advanced technology has resulted in many operations being possible, which could not have been performed before. Similarly, many once major operations are now being conducted as day-case surgery through much smaller incisions via minimally invasive surgery or key-hole surgery or as it's often called.

More recently Natural Orifice Translumenal Endoscopic Surgery (NOTES) has generated significant interest in what has become a new frontier of surgery through natural orifices. Specifically, NOTES refers to surgical procedures that involve the passage of a flexible tube through a natural orifice, including the mouth, rectum and vagina and where subsequent incisions are made in intra-abdominal or intra-thoracic organs. It appears to be safe and is likely to soon replace much of classical cancer surgery in certain parts of the body.

The aim of cancer surgery is to remove the whole tumour whilst leaving behind as much normal tissue as possible. The cancer surgeon has to perform a fine balancing act. The tumour must be removed in its entirety for the operation to be a success. But if at the same time too much normal tissue is removed with the tumour, the patient may have serious problems later. Progress in cancer surgery has come from knowing confidently how much tissue needs to be removed. New diagnostic imaging tests now allow us to predict far more precisely than even a decade ago the actual site of the cancer and its spread.

Surgery – what you need to know
- The aim of cancer surgery is to remove the whole tumour leaving behind as much normal tissue as possible.
- There is a great deal of controversy about the best type of surgery for different cancers. Are you sure you understand the alternatives?
- The period of convalescence after surgery varies enormously depending on the amount of collateral damage to normal tissues.
- Understand from the surgeon in advance the potential side effects.
- Do not sign a consent form for the operation unless you are entirely satisfied you understand what is happening.
- Explore alternatives to radical surgery – are there less extensive procedures that can be carried out. Join a relevant patient advice group
- How good is your surgeon – how many similar procedures does he or she do each year and what are the results like? Does he or she publish in medical journals and go to relevant conferences? The peak age for surgeons is 45–55 years. Younger surgeons may not be so experienced and older ones may get doddery.

Radiotherapy
Radiotherapy works by targeting ionising radiation directly at the cancer cells to damage and destroy them. Radiotherapy can cure many cancers by destroying the tumour or stopping it from growing any further. It is often used before surgery to reduce the size of a tumour prior to removal or after surgery to destroy any cancer cells that may be left behind. In some patients the cancer cannot be cured, but radiotherapy can be used to slow its growth and to manage and reduce cancer symptoms.

It is important that radiotherapy is targeted accurately to minimise damage to surrounding healthy tissue, though previously healthy cells can usually repair themselves if given time to rest. It is therefore equally important that the dose and timing of treatment are precisely calculated and monitored to allow healthy cells to recover.

Radiotherapy can be administered using beams of radiation aimed at the tumour from outside the body (external beam radiotherapy), or by introducing radioactive sources into the body. Radiotherapy is defined as the treatment of cancer and other diseases with ionising radiation. Ionising radiation deposits energy that injures or destroys cells in the volume of tissue being treated – the target tissue – and by damaging their genetic material, mainly the nuclear DNA, so making it impossible for them to reproduce. All cells possess DNA repair mechanisms, but cancer cells are streamlined for growth and their repair systems may not be so effective. Over 50% of cancer patients will receive radiotherapy at some point in their illness.

One of the greatest challenges is to minimize damage to normal cells by the delivery of an adequate dose aimed and timed accurately to destroy tumour cells and spare their normal counterparts. Although most of the media noise on cancer has been about access to high-cost drugs, there have been huge advances in radiotherapy. Similar post code lotteries exist around the use of the more sophisticated radiotherapy technologies. Better tumour imaging, new software imported from military systems and far more precision in delivery now allow pinpoint control of targeting with millimeter accuracy.

Selective tumour destruction can be achieved in two ways. The first is by the geographically precise deposition of radiation energy to the tumour. Modern tumour localising techniques involve sophisticated and often costly imaging systems such as CT (Computerised tomography), MRI (Magnetic resonance imaging) and PET/CT (Positron emission tomography). As all these images are computer generated it is possible to fuse them into one on a laptop screen – think of fusion cooking in restaurants. Powerful computer systems can be used to target the radiation beams precisely to the heart of the cancer.

The second selective mechanism is by the choice of the correct time, dose and scheduling of treatments to optimise the destruction of cancer cells whilst sparing normal tissue. A course of radiotherapy is usually fractionated – given in daily treatments (fractions) over a number of weeks. The mechanism of selectivity is complex and has been intensely studied over the last fifty years by radiobiologists. A simplistic view is that cancer cells have deranged radiation damage repair mechanisms and so are less well able to repair the damage caused by a fractionated course of treatment when compared to their normal counterparts. Over the last two decades the number of fractions given for treatment has been reduced. This is based on clinical trial data that demonstrate equivalent results and of course increased convenience for patients.

A linear accelerator (LINAC) is used to generate beams of ionising radiation by accelerating electrons in an electrical gradient down a linear tube for about one metre. The electrons, which by then are moving close to the speed of light, hit a tungsten target which converts their energy into heat and high energy, deeply penetrating X-rays. As they emerge from the LINAC they can be focused or collimated using specially cut metal-alloy blocks. More recently computer controlled, multileaf collimators have been developed consisting of small interweaving tungsten leaves that can be moved even during treatment. Pinpoint accuracy is now possible by using new techniques described below. Together, these two recently developed technologies allow the construction of easily reproducible plans to deliver a homogenous dose conforming to any possible shape, however irregular whilst continuously monitoring the position of the actual cancer within the delivered beams.

Intensity modulated radiotherapy – IMRT

IMRT uses cutting edge computer technology to produce complex, sculpted dose distributions which increase the dose to the tumour and decrease the dose to surrounding healthy organs. To deliver accurate radiotherapy it is imperative to ensure that the patient's position, and so the location of the tumour and surrounding tissues, is the same each time. A computer controlled, multi-leaf collimator in the output head of the LINAC allows the shape of each beam to be tailored to deliver the optimal high dose volume. The dynamic tungsten leaves in the collimator can change the shape of the beam even during the course of its delivery so increasing the number of possible shapes of the treatment volumes produced. So it is now possible to deliver a high dose of radiation to any shape desired – imagine a banana or a pear. When I began in radiotherapy, we could only do a ball or brick shape. Computers have revolutionized the whole area.

Image guided radiotherapy – IGRT

Traditionally, ink marks on the patient's skin have been used to position them on the LINAC couch for every treatment. The megavoltage treatment beam has then been used to produce simple images, on film or digital detectors, to image the bony anatomy and so verify the position of the treatment fields. This method assumes the position and shape of the tumour and critical surrounding normal tissues are fixed with respect to the bony anatomy, which is often not the case, and relies on planar megavoltage images which are not very clear. Both of these problems have been solved by the advent of IGRT in which CT imaging equipment, as used in diagnostic radiology, has been attached to the LINAC to produce images at the time of treatment.

IMRT/IGRT is now standard practice internationally for most treatments where cure is the aim. Randomised trials of its immediate precursor conformal therapy performed in the 1990's led to the widespread take up of that technique and randomised trials of IMRT carried out in recent years are continuing to gather new evidence. The results so far are very good.

Such trials are unlikely for IGRT, however, as it is not a change in treatment technique but rather a vast improvement in patient imaging and pre-treatment setup. The advantages of imaging the patient and correcting their setup before treatment seem obvious and it is unlikely that centres will be willing to randomise a control group to be 'treated blind' if IGRT equipment is available to them. A wide range of tumour types are now routinely treated with IMRT/IGRT in those countries with sophisticated radiotherapy services. These include lung, prostate, breast, head and neck and gynaecological cancers.

The patient is often likely to live for many years after treatment and so reducing the potential for long term collateral damage is essential. Not all patients may need IMRT as the anatomy of the tumour and normal tissue may permit clear discrimination without it. With palliative treatment, however, long term survival is unlikely and the delivered dose relatively low. IMRT may be indicated in special situations such as where a tumour is impinging on a vital structure, or the patient has been previously treated with radiation.

More recently MRI scanners have been attached to linear accelerators. This allows even more precision of dose delivery. The MR-LINAC, as such machines are called are far more expensive and require more staff to run. By taking an image between each fraction, adjustments can be made to the plan regularly so reducing the collateral damage caused by the irradiation of normal tissue. This is called Adaptive Radiotherapy.

Those that pay for your care have a tough choice. The costs of the more sophisticated planning and delivery technologies are up to four times that of conventional radiotherapy but will reduce as the numbers of patients treated increase. Is it worth spending more money on ensuring waiting time targets are met or developing better radical radiotherapy? Furthermore, independent sector providers geared to IMRT/IGRT are now coming on the scene. These may well offer much better services to private patients initially, so increasing the quality of private care. Such providers may be willing to provide a basic tariff for NHS patients – so resulting in a competitive marketplace in radiotherapy for the first time.

This all leads to a great variation in the quality of radiotherapy offered by different centres. The latest data from NHS England in 2021 still shows regional differences in the delivery of IMRT – from less than 60% to greater than 90%. And for IGRT the variation is even greater – from 40% to 100% even though all centres now have the necessary imaging equipment available. You need to find out what is available to you, and where. Talk to your consultant.

Precision radiotherapy may even be delivered as part of a top-up payment scheme now that such payments are permitted for cancer drugs. The provider landscape may undergo rapid changes throughout cancer care. There are clearly three financial pressures on those who pay for radiotherapy – improving access and delivering more fractions of conventional treatment; paying for more precise delivery systems in appropriate patients and dealing with requests for extremely expensive but specialist requests such as proton beam therapy. The dilemma is compounded by increasing awareness of precision radiotherapy delivery by patients.

Proton beam therapy
Magic rays that cure all cancers or expensive vanity projects of no real clinical value? The truth lies in between and depends on who you talk to.

The discovery of X-rays and gamma rays in the late 19th century led to a revolution in diagnosis and treatment of cancer. In 1903 William Bragg, a British physicist, discovered the very surprising behaviour of proton radiation. Protons are sub-atomic positively charged particles now produced by accelerating protons in a circular accelerator called a cyclotron. The advantage of protons lies in something called the Bragg Peak. This is the key to understanding why protons may be better for some patients.

The aim of radiotherapy is to deliver as high a dose as possible to the cancer but to spare as much as possible critically sensitive normal tissues around it. Certain organs are particularly sensitive – the spinal cord, base of brain, eye, intestine, liver and kidneys. The Bragg peak allows a more precise conforming of high dose to the cancer sparing any tissues downstream of the beam.

Before they reach the cancer, both proton and conventional radiation types have to make their way through the patient's skin and surrounding tissues. The photon, with no mass or charge, is highly penetrating and delivers a dose throughout any volume of tissue irradiated. However, most of the radiation is delivered only half a centimetre from the patient's skin, depending on the energy it was initially given. It then gradually loses this energy until it reaches the target. As tumours are almost always deeply located in the body, the photon actively interacts with outer healthy cells and drops only a small remaining dose of ionizing radiation on the deeper diseased cells. Moreover, as photons are not all stopped by human tissue, they leave the patient's body and continue to emit radiation as they leave the body. This is called the exit dose.

The proton, on the other hand, is a heavy, positively charged particle that gradually loses its speed as it interacts with human tissue. It is easily controlled and delivers its maximum dose at a precise depth, which is determined by the amount of energy it was given to it by the cyclotron. The proton is very fast when it enters the patient's body and deposits only a small dose on its way. The absorbed dose increases very gradually with greater depth and lower speed, suddenly rising to a burst when the proton is ultimately stopped. This is the Bragg peak. The behaviour of the proton can be precisely determined, and the beam can be directed so the Bragg peak occurs exactly within the confines of the cancer. Immediately after this burst of energy, the proton stops completely – its energy all spent. Proton therapy therefore allows to target cancers deep inside the body more precisely and spares critical surrounding tissue.

The problem is cost. Protons are nearly 2,000 times as big as electrons. Accelerating electrons down a long, straight tube is how conventional linear accelerator (LINAC) based radiation is produced. But protons require far more energy to get them moving. So a cyclotron is used accelerating them round and round in circles getting faster and faster. These are large and expensive bits of kit costing up to £100m with another £25m for the building to house them. Recently costs have fallen, and a compact model can be bought for a cool £25m. This compares with £2.5m for a conventional radiotherapy machine. So, what's the excitement?

Proton beam therapy is currently horrendously more expensive than conventional LINAC based radiotherapy. With legacy systems the cost ratio of protons/conventional is nearly tenfold. With compact systems and adequate numbers of patients this falls to below two. As the price differential diminishes, it is likely that there will be increasing demand of protons where the planned target volume can be achieved with greater critical normal tissue sparing by using protons.

It is now unlikely that there will ever be large scale randomised clinical trials but rather a pre-treatment comparison of proton versus conventional radiotherapy in individual patients using predetermined metrics of plan quality. This assessment would be made objectively by treatment planning software system. Payers, both governments (such as the British NHS) and insurers will use these criteria to assess the value of proton to an individual patient using the equation:

$$\text{VALUE} = \frac{\text{QUALITY} + \text{ACCESS}}{\text{COST OF TREATMENT}}$$

This formula applies to any service whether it's a cup of coffee from a café or a complex cancer treatment. Such analyses will determine the level of the therapeutic plateau in the relationship of cost to clinical outcome gain. Unfortunately, a literature review can only be of limited value in predicting demand for protons and how market forces will interact with evidence-based studies in the minds of payers. Furthermore technology shifts with a steady increase in the quality of imaging, planning and delivery of both protons and conventional radiation makes studies carried out even three years ago less relevant.

The use of protons is likely to be indicated for three groups of patients.

1. Hard indications – mainly children with spinal cord and brain tumours.
2. Cancer types where a significant proportion of patients are likely to benefit – lung and prostate – through reduced long term side effects.
3. Patients where the anatomy of the tumour and critical normal tissues favours a dose distribution with protons. This could be of any cancer type or site where radical radiotherapy is being proposed. That means the radiation is being given with the aim of eradicating the cancer, so curing the patient.

Calculating the demand for protons and the number of machines needed for a given population is difficult. The literature is weak, consisting mainly of calculations based on committee opinions of likely future indications and dovetailing this with past epidemiology from cancer registries. There are six such studies identified. There are no randomised controlled trials and these are unlikely in the future. A major problem in any analysis is the gradual improvement the dose distribution achievable by conventional linear accelerator delivered radiation over the last decade. Comparisons to conformal therapy are not so relevant in an era of IMRT (Intensity modulated radiotherapy), VMAT (volumetric modulated arc therapy also called RapidArc), SABR (Stereotactic ablative radiotherapy) and 100% IGRT. These acronyms are the new buzzwords of the radiotherapist and allow for much greater accuracy in radiation delivery.

The most informative study was carried out in Boston, USA. Here a comparison was made of proton versus conventional plans retrospectively in all patients treated over a one-year period in 2008. 1042 patient plans were analysed and scored. This allows the potential proton utilisation scenarios as a percentage of total fractions delivered to be calculated. The two main weaknesses of this study are the use of conformal therapy and not IMRT as a comparator and the optimistic committee judgement in an academic US centre to assess percentage of proton utilisation. They concluded that 17% of all patients would have benefited from the use of protons. Several proton demand studies have been carried out. Not surprisingly the results differ between countries with the USA at 20%, Sweden 16%, Italy 13%, France 12%, Holland and the UK 10%.

Let's look at what this would mean for the UK. The estimated demand for proton machines is based on a capacity per unit of 500 patients annually (20 average fraction delivery time, 25 fractions per course, 12 hour working 6 days per week). At a 10% level the machine requirement for the UK is therefore 18 machines. If an 18 hour double shift working day is implemented treating 750 patients annually then the requirement could be reduced to 12 machines.

Is this achievable? So far two machines have been very slowly being installed by the NHS – one at University College Hospital in London and the other at Christie Hospital, Manchester. The money was allocated in early 2011 and there has been more talk than action. Large legacy machines have been chosen costing £80m and requiring 80 staff each to run them. Varian, the company that manufactures them has merged into Siemens – a much larger medical equipment manufacturer. They have decided to get out of the proton business.

The compact models made by competitor IBA in Brussels, Belgium were installed by private sector providers but for NHS use cost less than £25m and require only 20 staff. That means the cost per single treatment will be far more expensive in the NHS installations. If everything is taken into account, the UCLH/Christie true cost for a single day of treatment will approach £5,000 whereas the compact model cost will be less than £1,500. And remember that most patients will need at least 20 treatments every day for four weeks.

We know that the average quality of British radiotherapy is poor with a huge need to upgrade the routine delivery machines many of which are more than a decade old. Capital is short as the NHS heads for a £30bn deficit by 2025. Imaginative new ways of funding state of the art cancer care are urgently needed in the UK and in many other countries. The disease is rapidly rising in incidence as populations get older and we really need to improve the care we give to all our patients. In chapter eight we will examine how to ensure you are getting the best quality of radiotherapy available even if you have to travel further for it.

For the last five years I've been the medical director of a proton network in the UK at Rutherford Cancer Centres. It's a very sad story but I have to confess being closely involved. In 2015 we obtained funding to build four proton units in the UK. We selected Newcastle, Reading, Newport South Wales and Liverpool as our sites. We built the units having raised over £200m of investment capital. All was going well until earlier this year when financial problems hit. The NHS avoided using us for protons although they were willing to use our linear accelerator and chemotherapy areas.

The reasons are simply for rationing although nobody will admit that. It can't be that the decision makers in the NHS are right and those in all other European countries are wrong. Spain has just ordered eleven of the same machines Rutherford uses. Yet the NHS says the two machines at Christie, Manchester and University College Hospital London are all they need and will not to buy treatments from elsewhere. All sorts of reasons were given but basically it was a rationing exercise. The four Rutherford centres are currently empty and idle. They do contain fantastic equipment at the time of the greatest backlog in cancer for my career. This has been a great personal disappointment and we're desperately trying to negotiate the reopening. But the current owner Equitix, an infrastructure property investor, wants a generous rental agreement underwritten by the NHS who have no spare cash. It's broke. Hopefully by the time you read this a workable solution will be found and protons will be available to both NHS and privately insured patients for a range of cancers.

Your radiotherapy checklist
- When will the treatment be planned?
- How long will planning take?
- When will the treatment start?
- How many treatments will I have?
- How long will they last?
- Will it be done using IMRT/IGRT, an MR-LINAC or proton?
- How much flexibility is there about the time of treatment each day?
- What are the immediate side effects and what should I do about them?
- Is there anything I should avoid: sunbathing, swimming, washing?
- How often will I see a doctor?
- What happens when I complete treatment?
- Who will organize and supervise any necessary follow up?

Chemotherapy

Chemotherapy drugs target cancer cells to destroy them and stop them dividing further. There are many types of such drugs, some based on natural plant compounds and others using man-made chemicals. Your oncologist will design a treatment plan specifically for you, incorporating the latest advances in chemotherapy to achieve the best treatment results. Chemotherapy is often used in combination with other treatments such as radiotherapy and surgery.

The chemotherapy treatment and drugs you are given depends on the type of cancer you have, where the cancer is situated, the type of cancer cells and whether or not the cancer may have spread.

When we look back at the history of oncology, we are humbled by the enormous power of some of the things we've been able to do. Patients with testicular cancer, Hodgkin's lymphoma, even breast and colon cancer patients for whom we can now offer significant life-changing intervention with chemotherapy. We are also humbled by the limits of what we've been able to achieve and the frustrations we've experienced. There are a number of phrases that we've been exposed to over the years that reflect the kind of journey it has been: single agent, combination therapy, schedule dependence, dose intensity, dose density, big dose, small dose, killing cells, regulating cells and more recently highly specific targeting, dirty specificity and off target effects. Great buzz words but the key is improvement in outcome for individual patients.

There are four key questions for doctors and politicians:

- What is the biological model for giving chemotherapy?
- What are our measures of success to be – the end points and the surrogates?
- What are our therapeutic goals?
- How does that model take into account our respect for the person and our societal values including the cost?

Cancer can be treated effectively by surgery and radiotherapy or both together but only when it is localized to a particular site of the body and the treatment is targeted accordingly. But, as we've seen, the main problem with cancer is that it spreads, first along the lymphatic channels, the nearby lymph nodes and then into the blood stream and beyond into other organs. Surgery and radiotherapy can only deal with local disease. When spread has taken place the treatment which must be systemic. That means it has to circulate around the whole-body system reaching any sites wherever the cancer cells may have spread to. The next chapter examines how cancer drugs were discovered and how they work.

Chapter Seven: Modern cancer drugs

Their discovery and clinical trial

Until 1943 there was no known drug effective against cancer. But all sorts of compounds had been tried. In the First World War mustard gas was used in the trenches but although it caused severe injury and death its mechanism remained unexplored. During the Second World War, the US military began experimenting with new chemical weapons. They came across the alkylating agents: drugs which bind and damage DNA in every cell. These drugs completely destroy the mechanism whereby DNA produces its message and replicates. Basically, it screws up the genetic machinery of cells. The first of these agents was nitrogen mustard and many other related compounds were subsequently discovered.

On a dark early December night in 1943 the Allied fleet consisting of British, American and French battleships were tied up neatly in Bari Harbour in Southern Italy. Unexpectedly, the Germans identified their location and bombed the harbour persistently during the night. It was a complete surprise. One of the major American battleships, the *John Harvey*, was shelled below the water line and sank into the murky waters of the harbour. Twenty-one ships were sunk and over a thousand people killed by the explosions. Some survived having floated in the sea for hours after the attack. Their rescuers noted that there was thick oil coming from some canisters in the *John Harvey* which had cracked, releasing their lethal contents into the sea around the sunken boat. Everything was shrouded in secrecy. The nitrogen mustard in the canisters was not listed on the ship or port manifest. Neither the Captain of the *John Harvey* nor the Bari Harbour Superintendent were aware of the lethal cargo intended for possible use as a chemical warfare agent.

I've been to Staithe 42B at Bari – the place where the John Harvey was moored. It was a beautiful autumn day. The blue sky and gentle wind gave a peaceful ambience to what had been a scene of destruction all those years ago. At the harbour entrance a plaque commemorates those who died that night and tells the story of the discovery of the cancer drug. But some dispute that the incident played any part claiming it was all a public relations ploy by the US to deflect the use of chemical warfare agents against the rules of the Geneva Convention at the time.

A week after the bombing at Bari the soldiers and sailors exposed to the oil suddenly dropped their white blood counts precipitously. This led to Dr. Lewis Goodman, an American pharmacologist working in the naval hospital in Bethesda, Maryland at the time. He had the idea of giving patients with lymphoma and leukaemia who had a high white count caused by cancer, nitrogen mustard intravenously. The first paper dealing with the dramatic response to this type of chemotherapy was written up in the *Journal of the American Medical Association* in March 1944. This marked the beginning of chemotherapy for cancer. There were many unpleasant side effects: severe nausea, vomiting but the shrinkage of the tumour was dramatic in several patients. Some did not respond, and all eventually relapsed because the cancer became resistant to the effect of the drug. But an effect had been seen. The search was now on for more anti-cancer drugs.

Since 1945 more than 500 cancer drugs have been discovered and are used regularly in clinical practice around the world. The drugs work through a whole range of mechanisms, some of which still remain unclear. Some drugs still work at the level of DNA, preventing it from being copied, a vital process in cell division. These drugs distort the DNA structure and prevent the attachment of the enzymes necessary for it to copy itself and enable two cells to be produced from one. Other drugs deplete the cell of the building blocks of DNA so that fewer raw materials are available for its replication. Still other drugs prevent binding of enzymes to produce ribonucleic acid (RNA), the message made in translating the thread of life, vital for the production of proteins, the executive molecules of the cell. A number have been discovered completely by accident. For example, the periwinkle plant, probably to be found as a weed in your garden, produces a family of drugs collectively known as the Vinca alkaloids – vincristine and vinblastine. These block cell division by preventing small bundles of intracellular muscles from pulling chromosomes apart at the time of cell division.

Cancer drug discovery
The majority of the most successful cancer drugs today were mostly discovered completely by accident. But the landscape is changing with the major inroads made on understanding the molecular defects that cause cancer. In the 1950's the National Cancer Institute in Washington, the largest cancer research hub in the world, embarked on a very ambitious programme of testing a whole range of substances. Scientists collected chemicals from all over the world, from all sorts of sources and tested them for their ability to kill cancer cells growing in test tubes. This programme uncovered a variety of chemical structures, which we

still use to this day. More than a million compounds have now been screened and vast data banks collected and archived.

There are far more romantic stories about the discovery of anti-cancer drugs. Several pharmaceutical companies developed programmes to search for new drugs in fungi and algae looking for a repeat of the famous penicillin story of Alexander Fleming. High above the Adriatic Sea in Northern Italy was an old tower built in medieval times. The tower itself is still a crumbling ruin overgrown with moss and ivy. Samples of bacteria were taken from this beautiful tower and a drug which interfered with DNA by inserting itself within its bases was identified. This drug was found to be remarkably effective in controlling breast cancer, Hodgkin's lymphoma and a number of other tumour types. The drug is known as doxorubicin but was given the brand name Adriamycin as it had been discovered on the Adriatic coast.

Even more exotic is a set of drugs used in kidney cancer treatment called mTOR inhibitors. mTOR stands for mammalian target of rapamycin. These growth control molecules were discovered by the purification of the antibiotic rapamycin from a bacteria found on Rapa Nui, the aboriginal name for Easter Island in the South Pacific.

The discovery of cisplatin, commonly used for testicular cancer, sarcomas and gynaecological cancer is another interesting story. In the early 1960's an American scientist, Bill Rosenberg, was interested in the ability of electrical fields to inhibit bacterial growth. He was a pure scientist working in a laboratory with no intention whatsoever of developing new anti-cancer agents. His experimental system was relatively simple.

He grew bacteria in a small dish and measured how many would grow in a defined period of time. He then inserted two electrodes and passed an electric current between them. He noticed that the growth rate of the bacteria diminished when the electric current was switched on. Initially he came to the conclusion that electric current inhibited bacterial cell growth. Being curious, he performed the following experiment. He took fluid from the bacteria which had been inhibited by the passage of an electric current and added it to fresh bacteria. Much to his surprise, he found that the growth rate for the second batch of bacteria was also diminished even though no electric current had been passed through them. A substance was clearly produced by the passage of electricity, which inhibited cell growth. This substance was found to be a soluble platinum compound produced by the passage of electricity through the electrodes during the experiment. Although platinum is familiar as a shiny silvery metallic solid, its organic form is a white crystalline powder which forms a clear solution. Cisplatin was the first of a series of platinum containing complexes, which were found to have considerable effect on particular cancers. A chance observation had thus given rise to an interesting new group of anti-cancer drugs.

But our classical older cancer drugs have profound side effects. The reason for this is that tumour cells and normal cells have very similar structure and function. This means that any drug that reduces cancer growth will inevitably also affect normal cells. This means that many cancer drugs have powerful side effects because of normal tissue damage. That is why they are usually only prescribed and monitored by those doctors that specialize in their use. Anti-cancer drugs inhibit cell turnover generally and so the most rapidly dividing cells in the body – the bone marrow, the lining of the intestine, the stomach, the skin and hair follicles – are the most severely affected.

In the skin, itching can occur, and hair loss is common. Some drugs are more notorious for causing hair loss than others. Adriamycin is the most likely drug to have this effect. There are ways of reducing hair loss by putting elastic bands around the scalp or cooling the scalp with an ice cap during the period when the drug is given. Basically, this causes the little blood vessels to contract so reducing blood flow and thus drug entry. None of these methods are completely effective but they do improve the results. The effects on the bone marrow result in a decline in the number of red cells leading to anaemia. White blood cells may fall leading to low resistance to infection. And the blood platelets – tiny factors in the blood vital for clotting – may also go down, leading to bleeding into the intestine and elsewhere.

Anaemia can easily be corrected by transfusion but thrombocytopenia (a drop in platelets in the blood) can result in abnormal bleeding into body cavities, which can be dangerous. To avoid the problems of bone marrow depression, patients having chemotherapy have a blood check to check their blood count and kidney function before each course of chemotherapy. There are ways of preventing bone marrow suppression but giving factors that stimulate the bone marrow to replicate and therefore produce a much more stable course for chemotherapy.

One of the keys to good cancer care is administering combinations of drugs in such a way as to maximize their effect on the tumour and yet minimise their effect on normal cells. In most cases the best way to do this is to give the drugs in large doses at intervals of three to four weeks. This enables the bone marrow and other critical tissues to recover in between. Tumour cells are not so well able to repair the damage caused by the drugs as their normal counterparts.

One of the major problems in the treatment of particular cancers is resistance to the drugs. It is thought that by giving several different drugs at the same time in larger doses, tumour cells will die before they have a chance to develop a resistance. Those cells resistant to one drug may not be resistant to another which acts through a different mechanism. This important aspect is the key rationale for combination chemotherapy. The other advantage is that the side effects of different drugs are not the same and therefore a dose of one drug is not necessarily limited by that of the other. This enables relatively higher doses of each to be given than were possible with a single agent.

One side effect that is often neglected by those caring for cancer patients is the psychological effect of repeated hospital visits often with much waiting around for the results of tests such as blood counts. Better organisation of cancer services can avoid these problems. Nausea and vomiting are now much less of a problem as we have very powerful anti-sickness drugs given before a patient first attends. One of the difficulties is what's called anticipatory vomiting, which arises from the association and experience of receiving chemotherapy.

It is explained by the phenomenon called conditioned reflexes. Pavlov, a pioneering Russian psychologist, studied salivation in dogs. He noticed that when dogs were given meat, they would salivate and drool if they were hungry. He always rang a bell before giving them the meat. After a period of time, the dogs would salivate in response to just hearing the bell, even though no meat was around. This process is called conditioning and we are all susceptible to it. An extreme example of conditioning occurred to a colleague of mine when shopping in the supermarket. A patient whom he was giving chemotherapy in the hospital saw him across the aisle and suddenly vomited. This was a vivid demonstration of conditioning.

Vomiting when undergoing chemotherapy can often become conditioned. The rationale for giving anti-sickness drugs alongside chemotherapy is that the first unpleasant experience of vomiting can be prevented, and so serious vomiting is less likely to take place later. In extreme cases, a patient can actually start to feel sick when they see anything associated with chemotherapy. If you are about to have chemotherapy, make sure you are fully covered with anti-sickness medication with each cycle of treatment.

Clinical trials

Much of the treatment given for cancer is based on assumptions and the accumulation of previous experience. Nevertheless, accepted therapies have not always been tested against alternatives and consequently much of the practice of oncology is not fully tried and tested. Clinical trials are necessary to determine whether new drugs are effective or whether when offered in combination they have fewer side effects than alternatives with the potential for destroying tumours. Clinical trials are an essential part of anti-cancer treatment.

Clinical trials on cancer drugs are divided into three phases. A phase I trial tests the dose and side effects of a new drug in around 20 patients. The first few patients may be given a very low dose – often far too low to see a good effect. But it's an essential process or otherwise lots of people may get dangerous side effects. Once a safe dose is established the study moves to Phase II. Here a set dose of a new drug possibly in combination with other established drugs for a particular cancer type is given to a series of patients carefully selected so that their cancer activity can be measured by a blood test or imaging. In this way the beneficial effects of a new drug can be seen quickly. 40–50 patients are usually enrolled. The last and most expensive component of a trial is Phase III when the new drug is compared usually in a randomised way to the best existing treatment available. Such studies are large, multicentre and usually international. A typical Phase III study may have 1,000 patients randomised to have 500 patients in each arm.

If the results are positive the drug company will go with the data to the regulators who will approve the drug for sale. The world's three main regulators are the Food and Drug Administration (FDA) in Washington, USA; the European Medicines Agency (EMA) in Amsterdam, Netherlands and the Pharmaceutical and Medical Device Agency (PMDA) in Tokyo, Japan. All countries have some sort of drug regulatory agency, but many just look at what the big three are doing. These agencies approve a cancer drug for sale for a specific indication – for example breast cancer. This indication is called the label for the drug and its wording is hotly contested by the manufacturer to boost sales. Increasingly many cancer drugs are used off-label – for cancers where the clinical trial data is not yet proven. Drugs and usually all clinical care in a trial are provided to patients for free. With off-label use the customer or the health system has to pay. This can cause tension as patients not unreasonably feel that they should be given all drugs that are likely to work against their cancer for free as part of their care.

If you are asked to join a clinical trial, remember it is purely voluntary and there is no obligation. You are also at liberty to ask to be removed from the trial at any point if you are not happy about your treatment. A consent form will require your signature and a full explanation of the study will be given. The trial will have been approved by a hospital ethics committee consisting of doctors and laypeople. Above all the ethics committee will decide whether the new treatment proposed is likely to be as effective as existing care. If this is not confirmed by the results, there is a fail-safe system for stopping the trial at any point and switching to conventional treatment. As well as contributing to future knowledge, participating in a clinical trial brings other dividends.

You will be more closely monitored and perhaps have more frequent checks of health and wellbeing than if not on the study. Most objections from patients to entering a trial arise because of simple misunderstandings. Be sure you know exactly what is being tried and why. It may not simply benefit you, but many others may benefit as a result of you taking part. And there is one consistent feature of well conducted trials – patients get better care as it is closely monitored. Things just don't get forgotten. Ask your GP and your oncologist about available trials relevant to your condition.

Where's chemotherapy going?

If we look at the results of chemotherapy now, we are often really deluding patients and ourselves of its benefit much of the time in those that have widespread cancer. We are very up-front about the word cancer but when we give chemotherapy for advanced disease, we're not so up-front about what it really means in terms of benefit. If you have cancer of the pancreas and are on second line chemotherapy for example, there's really no chance of surviving more than a year and yet we simply don't tell patients this. It's interesting to see how patients that doctors are ask far more pertinent questions about potential benefit and often decide to call it a day rather than continue to the end.

There are three groups of cancers in terms of the success of chemotherapy. In the first we can achieve a high percentage of complete response and a high cure rate. In the second where we have a high complete response rate – the tumour disappears completely – but the cure rate is low. In the third group chemotherapy is really not very beneficial at all giving just a few months extension of life. The problem with chemotherapy for advanced disease is that the good group contains less than 5% of all patients with cancer. If we look back at the last thirty years, the only disease in my professional lifetime that has shifted groups very significantly is testicular cancer. If there are going to be improvements, we'd expect to see some shifting of disease from the poorer to the better groups. That would be the clearest signal of success.

There's so much excitement about chemotherapy now based on human genome programme, bioinformatics, robots for high-throughput screening, computer drug design and whole platforms such as the kinases for which to create drugs. New biomarkers identifying pharmaco-dynamic end points are now available so we can measure if the drug is hitting on its target just by taking a sample of tissue from the patient. We now have surrogate end points and molecular signatures to predict response to different agents. A surrogate endpoint tells us within a day or so that the drug is hitting its target and working. The pathology of the future is not going to be about microscopic morphology – looking at the shape of cells and their architectural pattern, it will be about identifying the molecular constituents that rationally guide therapy.

There are currently just over 900 drugs in clinical trial for cancer of which about 500 are against very specific molecular targets. In 2020 there were 2,000 compounds and probably by 2025 there will be 5,000 compounds showing promise in the laboratory but not yet in use in the clinic. There are patterns evolving as the drug industry really has very little imagination. Everybody is developing drugs against the same targets. Currently the main theme is small molecules. They are easy to patent and simple to package either into vials for injection or as tablets in boxes. Monoclonal antibodies, cancer vaccines and gene therapy are on trial on a smaller scale, but the emphasis is very much on small molecules. There are only seven biological processes we need to consider:

- the cell cycle (the process of cell division)
- apoptosis (the natural way in which cells die)
- signal transduction (how growth signals are transmitted through the cell)
- angiogenesis (the growth of blood vessels into a cancer to feed it)
- inflammation (bringing immune cells into a cancer)
- invasion (the process by which cancer cells invade normal tissue)
- differentiation (that can make cancer cells stop growing and behave normally)

Nearly 80% of the entire global research portfolio of cancer drugs in development revolves around small molecules targeting the controls of these processes. The other approach is back to where chemotherapy began – the random screening of agents from natural sources. Taxol from the yew tree, vincristine from the periwinkle and doxorubicin from bacteria, all are products of systematic screening programmes. Most of the effective drugs we've got now come from natural sources and there are still huge ongoing programmes to look for more. We don't know where they're going to come from and it's very difficult to design a logical process. Rational drug design and random screening are the two most fertile hunting grounds for the future.

We have no idea how good future drugs will be. What we do know is that whatever comes out is going to be costly. McKinsey, the largest pharmaceutical consultancy in the world (based in New York), estimates that at the moment the cost of cancer drugs is $100 billion globally, of which about $70 billion is spent in the U.S. and $30 billion in the rest of the world. The US always dominates even though it is home to less than 5% of the world's population. McKinsey's prediction is a doubling in the market by 2025 to $200 billion based on increased numbers of cancer patients in an aging population and increased patient advocacy creating demand for new drugs. If we assume we get effective drugs into the clinic and it all pans out as planned then by 2030, the cancer drug market will be worth over $300 billion globally. This scenario of course depends on the drugs working and there being enough people willing to pay. There's no Plan B for the drug industry.

The effective use of diagnostics will become a central component of optimal cancer treatment. Diagnostics can be divided into clinical imaging and sample analysis in the laboratory. The latter can be split into assays for specific molecules and more holistic measurements of RNA, protein or modified structures. Increasingly, drug developers are turning to sophisticated diagnostic technologies to guide patient selection for trials of novel agents. Diagnostic tools such as biomarkers, surrogates, functional imaging, and molecular signatures are becoming essential in guiding critical decisions in the development of novel anti-cancer agents.

A cautionary word on how drugs are named. When being developed by clinical trial they are assigned a code which identifies the drug and the company involved eg. ZD 1839. The chemical name, in this case gefitinib is then turned into a generic name. The assignment of generic names to pharmaceuticals in development is an important prerequisite to marketing a drug. The United States Adopted Names (USAN) Program assigns generic names to all active drug ingredients. Outside the United States, the World Health Organization (WHO) publishes recommended International Nonproprietary Names (INN) for active drug ingredients. Consequently, the generic names inside and outside the United States differ only rarely, and these differences can potentially be very important. An example of a drug with two names is the substance known as acetaminophen inside the United States and as paracetamol internationally.

When approved by the regulatory bodies the company will assign a drug a trade name. Gefitinib became Iressa. This allows the creation of a branded product which will feature in all the adverts and public relations activities. So, all cancer drugs have two names – one generic which maybe complex eg ado-traztuzumab emtansine and a catchy, more pronounceable brand name – Kadcyla. Some generic names are totally obscure – try pronouncing inotuzumab ozogamicin or brentuximab vedotin after a glass or two of wine. The brand names are much easier Besponsa and Adcetris. The generic name is spelt with a lower-case initial letter whilst the brand name has a capital first letter. We teach medical students to use just generic names so that later in life they prescribe only generics. When the patent runs out the generics become much cheaper than the branded products, so this keeps the costs to the health system down.

The pharma industry wants you to use branded products as they make more money that way. I am sure you have seen advertisements on TV for Nurophen. If you go to a chemists shop the retailer wants you to buy that and not generic ibuprofen at a third of its price. The branded product is at the front of the display. It's a really crazy con trick and all doctors just buy generics for their families use – they are just the same stuff.

Molecular signatures and stratified medicine
Imaginative clinical assays, often using repeat biopsies of tumour and normal tissue, pose significant technical, logistical and ethical challenges. This area of research will drive much closer interactions between discovery and clinical groups, the creation of imaginative partnerships between academic centres and industry and the formation of specialist, diagnostic contract research organisations (CRO's). Multinational consolidated pharmaceutical companies are struggling to create new structures to encompass translational research and yet are under considerable time pressure to generate innovation forced by the

fact that the majority of high revenue cytotoxics will lose their patents and are now nearly all generic.

As we move into a molecular target-based future, cancer diagnostics will assume far greater importance in healthcare delivery. Initial treatment decisions are currently based on skilled histopathology and imaging studies to determine the type, grade and stage of the tumour. To this may be added immunohistochemical assessment of hormonal receptor status and prognostic markers such as c-erbB2 expression – the marker for the Herceptin target molecule. Yet histopathologists (pathologists who are expert at looking at tissues down a microscope) and their technical support staff are in short supply globally. This has driven increased laboratory automation at all stages from tissue handling through to image capture to reduce the costs, bring standardization and ability to perform tests far more speedily.

Diagnostic strategies based on sophisticated tissue analysis are now poised to radically change cancer management from the identification of people with a high risk of developing cancer through to the precise prediction of toxicity of a specific drug in an individual. Despite the hype genomics, proteomics and other holistic strategies are too vague to be used to guide drug development decisions in practice today. The large number of variables creates a bio-informatic nightmare. Achieving the goal of personalised medicine for cancer will require a revolution in diagnostics and the dawn of a new era in tissue analysis through classical quantitative immunohistochemistry.

Increasingly DNA found in the blood is being used to provide information about a tumour's behaviour. Circulating tumour DNA or ctDNA can be a rich source of information. This can be easily and repeatedly obtained by just a blood sample – no need for complex and sometimes hazardous repeat biopsies.

The traditional approach to cytotoxic drug development is not appropriate for many new agents for several reasons. Firstly, as their precise molecular mechanism is known it should be possible to develop a pharmacodynamic (PD) assay for their molecular effectiveness in patients. This can be used to determine the maximally effective dose for use in further studies. This approach will replace the classical phase I study which has in the past been used to evaluate the maximal tolerated dose. Although PD endpoints have been used for DNA binding drugs in the past specific relevant assays were simply not available.

Secondly it may not be possible to rely on tumour response in phase II as a guide to survival benefit. Many of the new agents will cause disease stabilisation and not shrinkage. Thus, it will be necessary to commit to expensive randomised phase III studies without having the confidence generated by a successful phase II programme. The key to success in this mechanistically based future will be the collection of far more data in the early phase of drug development using surrogates of both molecular target effects and clinical efficacy. Increasing emphasis on linking diagnostics to therapy will become an essential component of cancer drug development.

The holistic profiling of tumours using several technologies to determine its likely natural history and optimal therapy is possible. The beginnings of such correlations have been used in assays for the expression of specific gene products in increased, reduced or mutated form. Examples include erbB1, erbB2, ras and p53. The emerging technologies of genomics, methylomics, proteomics and metabolomics can produce enormous datasets to correlate with tumour behaviour patterns and response to different therapies. Although current data is fascinating, it will take several years before 'personalised medicine' becomes a reality for most cancer patients.

The next decade will bring novel technologies in all these areas together with increasingly sophisticated bio-informatic tools. There is now a great need for ethically collected fresh tissue – both normal and malignant – to develop novel assays and determine variation. The Human Tissue Authority in the UK was created to provide a well-defined legal framework for tissue donation after full consent. This provides an excellent ethical base for modern cancer research.

A toolkit for cancer drug development
The different components of an early development toolkit have different costs, risks and potential information yield. The investment payback will depend on how critical the information is to the successful development of drugs against a defined target. Thus biomarkers of molecular effect are a requirement for all drugs. Surrogate endpoints of clinical benefit are particularly important for drugs whose long-term administration is necessary to achieve either tumour stabilisation such as anti-angiogenic or anti-invasive agents where the cost in both time and effort of pivotal studies is immense. Success in achieving surrogate benefit here gives the confidence to commit long-term financial resource by effectively reducing the risk of failure and late-stage attrition.

Functional imaging studies which allow us to image the effects of a drug on the biochemistry of cancer cells in the body are particularly helpful where optimising the effect of a drug requires precise scheduling – cell cycle inhibitors and agents that cause cell death. By obtaining real time images of mitosis and cell death in patients, logical decisions to enhance selectivity can be made more easily. Some biomarkers may well be surrogates for clinical efficacy under certain defined conditions. Biomarkers have different levels of specificity. Some can be used for a range of drugs affecting a biological process such as angiogenesis – others may be highly specific for the effects of a single agent. The toolkit therefore consists of a series of drawers containing generic measurements for each category of a drug's action mechanism and a smaller compartment for the specific pharmacodynamic endpoint determination tools for an individual agent.

It currently takes an average of ten years for a cancer drug to reach the market from the identification of the lead compound. The sheer number of potential cancer drugs now becoming available and the change of emphasis to targeted molecular mechanisms will require a rigorous selection process during the early phase of clinical development. Timelines will get shorter. Over the next decade systematic programmes of cancer risk assessment will be established and cancer preventive agents will enter into the clinic. Novel surrogate endpoints will be essential to determine their benefit without waiting for a further generation of cancer patients.

One of the greatest challenges for an increasingly consolidated drug industry is to adapt to changing technology. The classical division of research departments into discovery and clinical is no longer optimal in this fast-paced area. Drugs entering the clinic need to come with validated biomarkers of their pharmacodynamic effect, surrogates for clinical efficacy and a plan to stratify patients for likely response. Effective organisation of translational science is the key to the future and yet a significant challenge.

Scientists are judged by the number of drugs getting out of the lab and into the clinic rather than how many are eventually brought to market and their commercial success. They are managed separately from clinical groups. Clinical departments are concerned with operational excellence in the construction and execution of clinical trials. The drive to keep research and development costs down has resulted in cross therapeutic area sharing of emerging laboratory technology which can adversely influence close collaborative working. That a problem exists has clearly been recognised by most companies as demonstrated by the willingness to experiment with their organisation.

Hormone treatment

Hormone therapy, also called endocrine therapy, involves the use of hormones, small molecules normally produced by the body, to treat certain cancers. Hormones act as chemical messengers that are produced by endocrine glands. These glands include the pituitary gland at the base of the brain, the thyroid gland in the neck, the adrenal glands above the kidney, the ovaries in women and testes in men. Many hormones control the normal growth of particular tissues, for example the female sex hormone oestrogen is produced in the ovary and stimulates the growth cells in the breast. Changes in the relative levels of different hormones control the normal menstrual cycle and changes in the ovary and lining of the womb during puberty and at the menopause.

Hormone treatment was discovered by a Scottish surgeon George Beatson. In 1896 in Glasgow, he removed ovaries from two young patients who had advanced breast cancer. In both women the disease stopped growing and indeed regressed. Though the tumours later returned, this was the first demonstration that changing the circulating levels of hormones could be effective against cancer. We now know that the removal of the ovaries leads to a fall in the level of oestrogen in the blood. The amount of oestrogen reaching the breast tumour is therefore less and the rate of tumour growth is reduced. Since Beatson's time, hormonal therapies have been widely used for other cancers arising in tissue susceptible to hormone influence such as the breast, prostate and uterus.

There are a number of ways in which the level of hormone activity can be influenced. The first is to destroy the endocrine gland that produces it. The gland can be removed surgically or given a dose of radiation high enough to stop it functioning and not to cause damage to surrounding tissue. It can also be tricked into switching off by giving a substance which mimics the naturally occurring trigger factor. Drugs can also be used to block the effects of the hormones produced by the endocrine gland. This has the advantage of being reversible but the disadvantage that the patient will need regular blood administration.

A whole range of hormone blocking treatments are available for both breast and prostate cancer and are remarkably effective without having any of the unpleasant side effects of chemotherapy. For hormones to work, they have to interact with the receptors in their target tissue. This can be likened to a key (the hormone fitting into the lock) to the receptor. If another substance fits the same lock but doesn't activate it, the hormone's effect can be blocked. Such drugs are called anti-hormones. The best example is tamoxifen, which blocks the action of oestrogen. Not all patients respond to hormonal treatment. Responses may be variable and slow even in cancers arising in the same tissue.

More recently a group of drugs called aromatase inhibitors have been particularly useful in older women with breast cancer. Even though the ovarian function ceases after the menopause, oestrogens are produced by skin, liver and other body tissues. The three drugs are anastrozole, letrozole and exemestane. They all work in the same way but have different side effects. These drugs are given orally and suppress the final pathway oestrogen production. Hormone treatment is usually used before chemotherapy in those patients that have susceptible disease, simply because it is less unpleasant, and chemotherapy can be kept in reserve if the cancer becomes hormone resistant.

Immunotherapy

Immunotherapy, also called biological therapy, is a type of cancer treatment designed to boost the body's natural defences to fight cancer. We've known that the immune system can recognise cancer cells as different from those of the rest of the body for many years but harnessing this recognition to bring about the targeted destruction resulting in cancer cell death has been much more challenging. Thousands of mice have been cured of cancer by using simple immunisation techniques, but these experiments have all been set up to favour the side of the immune system – after all, if it were that powerful why would cancer ever arise at all it should simply be wiped out in its infancy by such surveillance defence mechanisms?

There are several ways the science of immunology has been used to target cancer. Until five years ago it was thought that only a limited range of cancers would be susceptible. Melanoma, kidney cancer and lymphoma were always top of the list but currently we are seeing a remarkable change in direction with immune approaches being applied apparently successfully in a whole range of cancers including lung, brain and even breast cancer. The principle is to use materials either made by the body or in the laboratory to highlight target molecules or to restore immune system function by taking off its brakes. It's not entirely clear how most immunotherapy treats cancer. It may work simply by stopping or slowing the growth of cancer cells or by stopping cancer cells from spreading to other parts of the body. There are several types of immunotherapies including non-specific immune therapies, cancer vaccines, monoclonal antibodies and oncolytic virus therapy.

Non-specific immunotherapy

Most non-specific immunotherapy is a given at the same time as another cancer treatment such as surgery, radiotherapy, or chemotherapy. However, some can also be given as the main cancer treatment. The two commonest are interferon and interleukin 2.

Interferons help stimulate the immune system to fight cancer and may slow the growth of cancer cells. It's made in laboratories using recombinant pieces of DNA. The most frequent side effects include flu like symptoms, an increased risk of infection, rashes, thinning of the hair and tiredness which can be debilitating.

Interleukin 2 (IL2) help the immune system produce cells that destroy cancer. Again they are made in the laboratory. IL2 is used to treat kidney and skin cancers including melanoma. Common side effects include weight gain and low blood pressure which can both be treated by other medication. Some people may also experience flu like symptoms which can be severe.

Cancer vaccines

Cancer vaccines are another strategy used to help the body fight the disease. A vaccine exposes the cancer antigen to the immune system and triggers it to recognise and destroy any cell carrying that protein or related material on the cell surface. There are several types of cancer vaccine both for prevention and treatment.

A preventive vaccine is given to a person with no symptoms of cancer. It is used to prevent a person from developing a specific type of cancer. An example is Gardasil and Cervarix which are vaccines for human papilloma virus (HPV). This is known to cause cervical cancer and some other types including head and neck and anal cancer. In many poorer countries all children receive a vaccine that prevents infection from Hepatitis B virus. Long-term chronic hepatitis caused by this infection is known to be the main cause of liver cancer later in life.

A treatment vaccine helps the body's immune system to fight cancer. The system is amazingly complex and the antigens – the flags that distinguish cancer cells from normal – are very subtle. By training different components of the immune system to recognise and destroy cancer cells it may prevent cancer from coming back after surgery or radiotherapy. Many cancer treatment vaccines are still in development and only available through clinical trials.

Monoclonal antibodies

When the body's immune system detects something harmful it produces antibodies – proteins that fight infection. Monoclonal antibodies are a specific type of therapy made in the laboratory designed to attach to specific proteins usually on the surface of a cancer cell. Such therapies are highly specific, so they do not affect cells that do not have that protein on their surface. Monoclonal antibodies can be used in cancer as in various ways to allow the immune system to destroy cancer cells.

The immune system doesn't always recognise cancer cells as being harmful and this is one of the ways that cancer can grow and spread. Researchers have identified the Programmed Death (PD1) pathway as being critical to the immune system's ability to control cancer growth. By blocking this pathway with PD1 and PD L1 (Programmed Death Ligand 1) antibodies can stop or slow cancer growth. Such immunotherapy drugs are called checkpoint inhibitors because they interrupt an important part of the immune system. Examples are ipilimumab (Yervoy), pembrolizumab (Keytruda), nivolumab (Opdivo) and many others with increasingly unpronounceable generic names.

Monoclonals can be used to deliver radiation directly to cancer cells. The treatment is often called radioimmunotherapy. The antibodies deliver radiation directly to cancer cells by attaching radioactive molecules to them. They can deliver high doses of radiation specifically to a tumour whilst leaving healthy cells alone. Examples of these include ibritumomab and tositumomab.

Monoclonals carry other drugs directly a sort of guided missile. Once the antibody attaches to the cancer cell the treatment it is carrying is then delivered. This causes the cell cancer cell to die without damaging of the surrounding healthy cells. One example is brentuximab for certain types of Hodgkin and non-Hodgkin's lymphoma. Another is trastuzumab emtansine, a treatment for certain types of breast cancer, that initially responds to the well-known monoclonal antibody Herceptin.

Oncolytic virus therapy

This is a new type of immunotherapy that uses genetically modified viruses to kill cancer cells. A relatively harmless virus is injected into a tumour. The virus enters the cancer cells and makes copies of itself. As a result, the cells burst and die releasing a cloud of tumour antigens.

This triggers the patient's immune system to launch an attack on all the cancer cells of the body that have the same antigen. The virus does not enter healthy cells.

In 2015, the first oncolytic virus therapy was approved to treat melanoma. The virus used in the treatment is called talimogene or T-Vec. This is a genetically modified version of the herpes simplex virus that causes cold sores. It is injected directly into the melanoma lesions and generates widespread immune destruction of melanomas all over the body. Patients receive a series of injections until there are no lesions left. Side effects include fatigue, chills, fever, and flu like symptoms. Researchers are now testing other oncolytic virus for different types of cancer in clinical trials as well as in combination with other treatments such as chemotherapy.

Questions for your specialist
Talk with your doctor about whether immunotherapy may be part of your treatment plan. This is a very rapidly changing area. Consider the following questions:

1. what type of immunotherapy do you recommend?
2. what are the goals of treatment?
3. will immunotherapy be my only treatment?
4. how will I receive immunotherapy and how often?
5. what are the possible side effects both short and long term?
6. how will this treatment affect my daily life?
7. Will I have to pay extra to receive it?
8. what clinical trials in immunotherapy are open to me?

Chapter Eight: Some cancer types

Getting detailed information on services locally is vital

Breast cancer

Breast cancer is extremely common, with one in twelve women in Britain developing this type of tumour. That's over 50,000 women a year. There is a lot of controversy about the best way to treat breast cancer. There are really two problems. The first is how to treat the cancer in the breast itself and the second, how to reduce the risks of recurrence in other sites. Both involve a trade-off between damage to normal cells with the related side effects and the risk of the disease returning.

The problem with breast cancer is not dealing with the primary cancer but avoiding the consequences of metastasis. Metastasis just means "change of place" and is the process by which cancer cells break off and spread through the lymphatic channels or blood vessels and settle in other parts of the body. Tumours of the breast particularly like to form what are often called secondaries in the bone, liver, lung and less frequently the brain. The first line of metastasis is usually the lymph nodes in the axilla (armpit). Around 90% of patients developing early breast cancer will be cured of their disease. Those that are not cured develop recurrence and spread in other sites of the body. Most of the variation in treatment patterns is in dealing with the primary tumour.

Breast cancers tend to grow extremely slowly, many take up to five years to reach the size of one centimetre. The commonest way in which a woman notices a breast cancer is a painless lump often found while bathing or in the shower. Screening has increased the detection of early cancer although there is considerable controversy as to how worthwhile it really is. The problem is not that it doesn't pick up breast cancer, it also picks up a lot of minor abnormalities that really do not need to be detected and have no consequences for the life of the woman. This creates a huge amount of anxiety amongst the patient and their families and sometimes outweighs the benefit of a few months' earlier diagnosis.

The initial assessment of a patient suspected of having breast cancer includes a careful examination to assess the size, location of character of the primary tumour, together with evidence of spread of lymph nodes in the axilla and other areas around the breast. Some patients actually present with disease that has already spread, often to the bone. Sometimes they may ignore the ominous symptoms of a growing lump in the breast, and it can actually break through the skin creating very unpleasant infection around the breast. Investigations required to fully assess a patient with early breast cancer include a blood count, liver function tests, a CT scan of chest and abdomen and a bone scan. Other types of scanning are not routinely performed but may be requested if there have been abnormalities found on clinical examination or there are particular symptoms that give rise to the suspicion that the disease may have already spread. There are four treatments for breast cancer: surgery, radiotherapy, chemotherapy and hormone treatment.

Surgery

Until 1890 a crude wide excision of the cancer was the only procedure possible. In 1895 William Halstead, a pioneering American surgeon, developed an operation that was called the radical mastectomy. This became the archetype of many cancer operations. The primary tumour in the breast was removed, with surrounding tissue and in contiguity with the regional lymph nodes and underlying muscle. This operation was subsequently modified to reduce its cosmetic impact.

Over the last two decades the thrust has been towards more conservative surgery. Instead of performing a mastectomy the tumour alone is removed often with a one- or two-centimetre margin and the patient given postoperative radiotherapy. This approach gives a better cosmetic result with no evidence of an increased rate of local recurrence or poorer survival when compared with the more aggressive surgical procedures. It is not always possible to use this conservative approach. For example, if there is a large tumour in a small breast where its removal would result in a very poor cosmetic appearance and similarly if there are several tumours in the breast which does occur in about ten percent of women making mastectomy necessary. Alternatives are always discussed with patients, and they form part of the decision-making process. Nobody is compelled to have surgery or indeed any cancer treatment.

Radiotherapy

Radiotherapy is used in conjunction with surgery to prevent the disease coming back within the breast. It is important that it is planned carefully and delivered using advanced equipment preferably with IMRT and IGRT. We know that the long-term results of surgery and radiotherapy can be excellent. However, if radiotherapy is given using old fashioned techniques fibrosis, then other late side effects occur caused by damage to normal tissue surrounding the tumour's bed. Because of the breast's unusual shape in three dimensions and the inability to use a template because of variation between women, determining the correct technique for irradiating an individual breast is a very skilled process.

Chemotherapy

Chemotherapy is used in two ways: as an adjuvant after surgery and for treating known metastatic disease. Adjuvant therapy is defined as the use of additional treatment given after apparently successful removal of all known disease detectable by clinical X-ray and other investigations. Breast cancer has provided an incredible test ground for many trials of adjuvant treatment in both chemotherapy and hormones that have been used in other cancers.

The concepts behind adjuvant chemotherapy are logical. At the time of the removal of the primary tumour access to any small areas of spreading cells will be good, the patient will tolerate even aggressive regimens as she is not in poor health because of the effects of large metastases. Remaining tumour cells should theoretically be sensitive to chemotherapy as they are dividing at their most rapid rate and finally there is good evidence from tumour model systems to support the role of adjuvant chemotherapy in preventing recurrence.

Adjuvant therapy began in 1965. Injections of chemotherapy were given immediately after surgery to reduce the ability of circulating tumour cells to get hold in distant organs. Although some benefit was seen the results were not startling initially. In the 1970's two large studies were published which showed that chemotherapy given for a year following surgery had a dramatic effect on long term survival. Over the years the drugs have changed and become much more tolerable. They are also given with supportive drugs to prevent sickness and other side effects have really revolutionised adjuvant treatment of breast cancer. Drugs that are commonly used in different combinations are 5-Fluorouracil, Epirubicin, Adriamycin, Cyclophosphamide, Herceptin, Docetaxel and Taxol.

Another strategy is to give neoadjuvant chemotherapy. Here the drugs are given before surgery. A great advantage is that the change in tumour size can be measured easily and so both patient and doctor know that the treatment is working. By drastically shrinking the tumour it can make surgery easier and more likely to remove the entire tumour.

The benefits of adjuvant chemotherapy are easy to determine by using the very educational website https://breast.predict.nhs.uk/. It represents the distillation of data from over 50,000 British women. You don't have to go through the tedium of registering and it's free and very good. Better still get your consultant to go through your options with you. You can really see how much or how little you will gain with adjuvant treatment with drugs or hormones. It's all about individual risk assessment. By using predict you can take charge and determine yourself what risks you are willing to take. It's exactly like going to a financial advisor to decide on what investments to make. In Britain, patients are not usually offered the chance to be involved. Grab the opportunity when you can – after all it's your life.

Over 80% of patients will survive following primary treatment of an early-stage cancer. However, for those where the disease recurs chemotherapy is also offered. A full assessment is made and if the recurrence has recurred outside the previously treated volume and is localized, then radiotherapy may be used instead. The same agents that are used for adjuvant treatment are given and the patient closely monitored after two or three cycles. The most important part of a management plan of the patient is to check that the tumour is actually disappearing when chemotherapy is given. This often takes two to three months and therefore a critical re-assessment is needed. A difficult clinical problem arises when chemotherapy is only partially effective. It is then up to both the physician and patient to balance the benefits in terms of tumour response with the drawbacks arising from the side effects of therapy. Remember, you're in the driving seat about what to do.

Hormone treatment
Hormone treatment like chemotherapy is used in both adjuvant and metastatic situations. A variety of drugs are available including Tamoxifen, Anastrozole, Letrozole and Exemestane. Sometimes these drugs have different trade names but they all act by suppressing the oestrogen drive for cancer cells by affecting the hormonal composition of the body. Most patients will have little side effects. Tamoxifen is much less used now but was the first anti-oestrogen drug to be discovered in the UK in the 1960's. It led to a plethora of other drugs that are in some cases more effective especially in women that have had their menopause.

There have been huge advances in the treatment of breast cancer over the last fifty years and this is reflected in the much better survival rate. There has also been an increasing trend for women to go to their doctors when they have any signs of early disease. This is good as it makes treatment much easier for both doctor and patient and the message has to be not to ignore a breast lump however innocuous it seems.

Prostate cancer

Cancer of the prostate is a common tumour and affects over 50,000 British men each year. Worldwide there is considerable variation with the lowest incidence being reported in Japanese men and the highest found in American Blacks. The cause is uncertain but an association with male hormone stimulation is postulated, although there is no direct relationship between sexual activity or serum testosterone levels. There is, however, a decreased incidence of prostatic cancer in patients with liver failure who may have higher than normal circulating levels of oestrogen.

The most confusing aspect of this disease is its natural history (at least in the early stages) and the relationship of a precancerous condition called carcinoma in situ to the invasive form of the disease. The progression of invasive carcinoma is through its growth within the prostate until it ultimately breaches the prostatic capsule to invade other organs in the pelvis. This is well documented. Invasive disease is associated with a progressively higher incidence of local lymph node spread and so a greater chance of distant blood-borne spread. This process by which cancer can leave the primary site in which it arose and go to other organs is called metastasis, meaning change of place. Favoured sites for metastatic deposits include bone, lung and liver, although bone is by far the commonest.

The tumour originates from the subcapsular part of the prostate, relatively distant from the more medial portion through which the urethra – the tube connecting the bladder to the outside world – passes. Therefore, the tumour has to be moderately large before local symptoms of obstruction to urinary flow are encountered in an age group which has a high incidence of symptoms from benign prostatic enlargement. The local symptoms related to the urinary system are thus hard to distinguish from benign causes, and presentation with painful bone metastases is not uncommon. Rectal examination in the asymptomatic patient will detect a significant proportion of these tumours, although transurethral resection of the prostate may fail to obtain malignant tissue. For this reason, many urologists prefer to obtain histological confirmation of disease by needle biopsy through the rectum – the back passage.

The incidence of prostate cancer increases with age, and the number of patients with small foci of malignant carcinoma in situ found at autopsy also increases with age. It is not clear whether these are inevitable developments of the ageing process and represent a stable form of disease, or whether all invasive carcinomas develop from one of these lesions. This has practical importance. Patients sometimes present with painful bones which subsequent investigation shows to be due to metastatic cancer. In a proportion of these patients, a small carcinoma of the prostate will also be discovered. Such metastases should not be assumed to have originated from the prostatic lesion.

The most important assessment for patients with carcinoma of the prostate is rectal examination. It will give information as to the extent and size of the prostatic tumour, the presence and absence of breaching the prostatic capsule and whether or not the pelvic side wall has been affected by tumour. The general condition of the patient should be noted and the presence or absence of any bone pain or tenderness to palpation recorded. Because this is a disease of elderly men, it is quite common to find unrelated medical conditions. Baseline investigations will include estimation of Blood count, alkaline phosphatase, liver function tests, chest x-ray, isotope bone scan, magnetic resonance imaging scan and the estimation of the PSA (prostate specific antigen). This latter protein shed from the cancer cell into the blood stream is not universally raised. When raised at presentation it may be a useful marker of disease and response to treatment. Several studies have now shown that rectal examination does not influence serum levels of PSA. However, a normal PSA does not exclude the presence of an active carcinoma.

Treatment
This will depend on the stage of the disease – how far it has spread within the prostate and also outside. There are patients whose disease is confined to the prostate and those whose tumour has breached the capsule and who have a high probability of distant disease. In the UK radical prostatectomy has never been a popular option; even for early-stage carcinoma it carries a high morbidity and significant mortality. Many patients are rendered incontinent following surgery and it is difficult to demonstrate any survival benefit. This is of course complicated by the uncertainty of the natural history of disease and the problems of predicting life expectancy in an elderly population. Robotic minimally invasive surgery is now available in most centres – ask your urologist if you are suitable.

For many men the best treatment is watchful waiting. This involves three monthly follow up with a PSA test and a repeat MRI every six months. There is no doubt we over diagnose prostate cancer, and many men will not develop any problems from it. We are getting better at sorting out those patients with small cancers that would benefit with early intervention.

Most oncologists in the UK recommend radical radiotherapy to the prostatic bed to deal with early-stage disease. There is good reason to believe that this can provide permanent local control over the tumour. Again, it is difficult to be certain what survival benefit is given. Similarly, the incidence of the later appearance of metastatic disease is not always influenced by the primary treatment. Pelvic radiation may be given in patients who have more advanced tumours, especially if there are local symptoms such as pelvic pain or bladder involvement. Before radiotherapy is started hormones may be given to shrink the primary cancer so reducing the volume and hence the side effects. New precision techniques such as IMRT (intensity modulated radiotherapy and IGRT (image guided radiotherapy) ensure pinpoint accuracy and greater efficacy. Sadly such treatments are not always available. You have to ask around. It is likely that proton beam therapy will have considerable advantage in around a third of patients receiving radiotherapy for prostate cancer – the results of clinical trials are now beginning to emerge. How the NHS will provide the service remains to be seen.

The treatment of metastatic disease from carcinoma of the prostate is controversial. It has been known since the 1940s that the administration of oestrogen is capable of causing regression of prostatic enlargement, both benign and malignant. Traditionally, this has been achieved through the administration of stilboestrol or by removing both testes which reduces testosterone secreting tissue and consequently increases effective oestrogen levels. Early studies using high doses of stilboestrol demonstrated an elevated incidence of cardiovascular mortality, and indeed in one trial the treatment group fared rather worse than the control group because of incidental cardiovascular deaths despite evidence of good tumour regression. For this reason, orchidectomy was the preferred choice of the first line therapy for metastatic prostatic carcinoma. However, more recent studies using lower dose stilboestrol showed good response rates with little cardiovascular toxicity.

More recently, synthetic oestrogen-like substances, such as fosfestrol have been found to be effective in controlling the disease. Gonadotrophin analogues such as luteinizing hormone-releasing hormone (LHRH) agonists are capable of affecting the disease progress by down-regulating testosterone production. Androgen-receptor blocking agents such as bicalutamide and flutamide are also being used. Most controversy revolves around the time at which such treatment should be offered. It is unclear whether first line therapy should be offered immediately on the demonstration of metastatic disease, or whether they are equally effective when symptoms arise, or whether they are equally effective when symptoms arise. Similarly, the protective effect of these procedures in the absence of demonstrable metastatic disease is not clear. Currently clinical trials are in progress to settle these questions.

Eventually the cancer cells mutate to become insensitive to the effects of withdrawing male sex hormones. At this point chemotherapy with docetaxel (Taxotere) is used. The key here is to monitor its effectiveness very closely by following PSA levels and using CT and MRI scans.

The prognosis is difficult to establish given that the population is elderly with a limited life expectancy irrespective of the cancer. In principle, it appears that those patients found at an early stage in the absence of metastases can look forward to a long natural history with appropriate treatment and are unlikely to die as a consequence of their disease. The average expectancy of life of a patient presenting with an invasive tumour is between 1 and 4 years, although this may well represent the normal life expectancy of the population. There is no reason to believe that age has any significance in terms of eventual outcome.

Several new drugs and vaccines are becoming available for treating patients whose disease has spread. These include abiraterone, MDV 3100 and alpharadin. They are all very expensive.

Determining prognosis is very difficult. In July 2009 I was asked to provide advice on the likely outcome of Mr. Al Megrahi, the "Lockerbie Bomber" who had prostate cancer. It all began with an unannounced visit to my office by a shadowy but charming fixer who floated between London, Tripoli and Washington. I had visited Tripoli in my previous role as Chief of the WHO Cancer Programme to try to resolve drug and equipment supply issues during the UN embargo and I was well known to the oncologists in Tripoli and helped them access cancer drugs.

Assessing a patient with prostate cancer seemed a routine task. It seemed reasonable for the Libyans to know how strong their case was for arguing for Mr. Al Megrahi's compassionate release. I had tea with Saif Gadaffi, the son of the President, in London at the Intercontinental Hotel in Park Lane to explain the strategy. We would take three doctors to Greenock Prison outside Glasgow to review all the clinical information. We agreed that we would be paid the NHS Litigation Authority standard rate for medico-legal experts. I hadn't envisaged the media storm that would erupt.

I visited the prison in July 2009 and met and examined Mr. Al Megrahi as well as reviewing his X-rays and notes. I discussed his case and its progress with his prison doctor to better understand the pace of his illness. Assessments of his condition had been made by at least nine specialists at that stage although only five had actually seen him in prison or hospital. Based on the evidence of rapid spread and progression of his cancer despite the correct treatment, I wrote a report which stated that on the balance of probability he would die at around three months assuming he would receive standard NHS care in Glasgow. Arriving at an exact prognosis in prostate cancer is impossible as there are always some surprisingly long-term survivors however bad the situation.

It is always difficult to convey the statistical chance of a specific medical event happening. There are an enormous number of variables involved. Death is ultimately caused by cancer causing the failure of a specific organ such as kidney, liver, lung or through a terminal infection. These are very unpredictable events. There are clues as to the pace of any cancer. These can be deduced from taking a history, from examining the patient and from reviewing a series of X-rays and blood tests. Then it becomes a value judgement of probability.

My report was submitted to the Libyan Embassy. At no time was it suggested by staff of the Libyan, US or British Governments that I should modify it. After his release in August 2009 the Scottish Office issued a statement that my report had arrived too late to be taken into consideration. "Their reports were not actually received by Scottish Government officials until four days after Dr. Andrew Fraser's report was submitted to the Justice Secretary, and therefore played no part in Mr MacAskill's decision on compassionate release". They had used their own medical advice, collated by Dr. Fraser, Head of the Scottish Prison Medical Service which must presumably concurred with mine, in forming the decision to release Mr. Megrahi on compassionate grounds.

It has been reported that I changed my mind on the prognosis subsequently. When asked by a reporter if it was possible that Mr. Megrahi could live another ten years my response was – "yes, it's possible, but highly unlikely". This answer was twisted into a statement that he would live another ten years. This was absolutely untrue.

In cancer medicine we often use survival curves to assess the benefit of new treatments. Clinical trials are carried out to determine whether a new drug has benefit compared to an old one. When a patient wants to know their likely prognosis, we now are very honest, always explaining the wide range of outcomes. But it's like trying to piece together the plot of a ballet after seeing just one still shot. Most people would die at three months but there is a very wide range with a long tail to the curve.

Conspiracy theories abound – I was shown the wrong patient, the X-rays and blood tests were faked, maybe he died shortly after his release or simply that we were all bribed to get the answer the Libyans wanted. I don't believe any of this. Subsequently, Mr. Al Megrahi had excellent care in Tripoli, until the tumultuous events that led to the end of the Gadaffi regime. Although it was unexpected that he would live for 3 years he was treated very aggressively with new drugs. His quality of life in Tripoli was very poor and he was in bed most of his last year of life.

Ironically, he was treated with abiraterone. This drug was discovered in Britain using Cancer Research UK charitable funding. It was given its license by the European Medicines Agency in September of 2011 and was not available to most patients on the NHS until 2018. It costs about £4,000 a month and the only way to get it on the NHS was through the Cancer Drugs Fund. Megrahi was also on a range of other therapies not available here.

I feel very sorry for any distress the whole episode caused for the families of the victims of the Lockerbie bombing. Maybe now, thirty years on, they can close a very painful and emotionally fraught chapter in their lives. The 25th anniversary of the event was marked by a very solemn service in Westminster Abbey.

Surprisingly few cancer patients actually ask for a specific prognosis. We always try to be as truthful as possible but within the limitations of the wide variations of the natural history of any cancer. The sad episode of the Lockerbie Bomber has taught me to be even more cautious than before – unusually good things can happen to cancer patients. In an age of molecular reductionism with magic bullets and personalised medicine with smart drugs, there are many things we still don't understand. We remove hope at our peril.

Colon cancer
Cancer of the colon is common in western countries. This has led to the

speculation that the western diet with its emphasis on refined foods of low fibre content has a part to play in the aetiology of this disease. Certainly in countries where the diet naturally contains large amounts of fibre it is a relatively uncommon tumour.

Clearly recognised predisposing factors include ulcerative colitis and familial polyposis coli. The latter is rare but important to recognise. In this condition polpys tend to appear in early adulthood and one or more will inevitably progress to frank malignant change unless treated. Because the number of polyps is so large, regular check-ups with either endoscopy or barium contrast x-rays are not practical, and most surgeons recommend elective colectomy leaving a rectal stump so the patient remains continent. This short stump can then easily be examined via the sigmoidoscope, and any polyps dealt with locally on a regular basis before invasive malignant change develops.

Cancers frequently arise in benign polyps. In both familial and isolated lesions the natural history is for epithelial metaplasia to form a polyp which gradually becomes less polypoid and more villous in nature. This can then become invasive by growing around the circumference of the bowel and will eventually penetrate directly through the bowel into the surrounding tissues.

The whole strategy of screening for colon cancer is based on this polyp to cancer transition. A small polyp occasionally bleeds, usually not enough to be noticed. But small amounts of haemoglobin from blood can be detected in the stool by a chemical. The current UK screening programme starts at age 60 and involves testing for occult blood in the stool. If the test is positive then a colonoscopy is offered. This involves passing a flexible tube into the rectum and through which the inside of the entire colon can be visualised and photographed. Furthermore, any polyps can be snared with a wire and removed. By removing benign polyps colon cancer can be prevented.

Once a cancer is established lymphatic spread to regional lymph nodes is common, although the lymphatic system does seem to have some arresting potential for the disease. Distant lymphatic spread is often associated with advanced cancer. The intestinal lining is rich in blood vessels and the portal system in particular readily transports metastatic cells into the liver. Liver spread is increasingly frequent with more locally advanced tumours. Depending on the position of the tumour within the bowel, it is also possible for seedling deposits to spread throughout the peritoneal cavity causing multiple nodules, which may lead to the formation of ascites – the gathering of fluid in the abdomen.

How it starts

The clinical picture produced by an early colon cancer will depend on its position within the bowel. Those on the right side tend to be relatively silent in the early stages, as the bowel contents here are soft and have no difficulty in passing through a narrowed pipe. A common presenting feature of right sided carcinoma is anaemia due to blood loss through the tumour surface into the gut. Patients with tumours on the left side. where faeces are more solid, tend to notice constipation, alteration in bowel habit, or frank bleeding. In general, anyone over 40 with a change in bowel habit, particularly associated with the passage of mucous or blood, should be investigated within weeks to exclude a cancer of the colon. Not uncommonly, secondary deposits in the liver result in jaundice, an enlarged painful liver or ascites (fluid in the abdomen causing swelling) as presenting features.

Physical examination is the most important first step to sort things out. Seventy five percent of tumours will be directly visible through a tube passed up the rectum – a flexible colonoscope, and around 50% can actually be felt on rectal examination. Other investigations include the detection of faecal occult blood and a CT scan. The features of a colon cancer are characteristic on X rays and CT scans and this may reveal more than one tumour, a factor which clearly influences subsequent treatment.

Treatment

Treatment of this cancer is largely surgical. The aim is to remove the tumour by wide resection, together with regional lymph nodes and usually involves a hemicolectomy. Even in the ill patient with obvious tumour spread, the best palliation is provided by surgery. Tumour left untreated will inevitably lead to obstruction and local pain. This can often be alleviated by bypassing the tumour and the formation of a colostomy. Other modalities of treatment have relatively little to offer early in this condition. In the case of pelvic tumours radiotherapy given preoperatively may produce good local reduction in the tumour size, making an otherwise inoperable tumour operable.

Radiotherapy has its part to play later in the course of this disease, when local recurrence may occur. Usually, this will present as pain, often within the pelvis or perineum. A short course of radiotherapy can give good palliation to this distressing symptom. Adjuvant chemotherapy may reduce the risk of spread. Neoadjuvant radiotherapy and chemotherapy can shrink tumours especially in the rectum so making surgery easier increasing the chances of normal bowel control afterwards.

Several drugs are effective at reducing the spread of cancer. The most common combination used in the UK is now FOLFOX. This contains three drugs: 5 Fluorouracil, Folinic acid and Oxaliplatin. The same combination can be used for patients with secondary spread. Sometimes the 5 Fluorouracil which has to be given intravenously is replaced by capecitabine (Xeloda) which is given as tablets twice a day. The combination of capecitabine and oxaliplatin is called CAPOX or XELOX. In about 30% of patients the tumour shrinks significantly, but drug resistance often supervenes. Another similar combination is FOLFIRI where the oxaliplatin is replaced by irinotecan. Putting everything together as in FOLFIRINOX is sometimes used but as you can imagine increasers the potential of serious toxicity.

There are two other rather expensive drugs known to prolong survival which can be added. They can be made available through the NHS but often are simply not mentioned. Ask if they are suitable for you. They are bevacizumab (Avastin) and cetuximab (Erbitux). They are not for everybody but it's up to you to ask about them.

Because of the propensity of these tumours to spread through the vein draining the intestine into the liver the use of 5-fluorouracil injected directly into the vein at the time of surgery has been investigated. The number of patients with subsequent liver metastases appears to be reduced, but there is little evidence of an overall improvement in survival.

The most likely avenues for progress in this disease include better screening and early detection, making it possible to initiate treatment at a much earlier stage of the evolution of the disease before dissemination has occurred and when surgery is much more likely to be successful.

Lung cancer

Cancer of the lung, more correctly known as carcinoma of the bronchus, is still the commonest cancer in Britain. It affects over 40,000 people in the UK each year. Despite its well-known association with cigarette smoking, increasing numbers of young people continue to smoke. There are several other causative factors, in some cases, directly related to smoking habits. These include a preponderance among lower socio-economic groups; a 4:1 male to female ratio, although this is changing with increased smoking among women; and a variety of occupational groups who have a particularly high incidence of this disease. These include workers in industries where exposure to radiation is common, such as the uranium mines of South Africa; those that have been exposed to asbestos in pipe lagging and roofing; and workers coming into contact with arsenicals in sheep-dips, vineyards and tobacco processing plants.

An increasing number of young women are smoking for reasons that are not clear. None of the covert advertising is aimed at them. The most plausible theory is that 12–14-year-old girls are obsessed by their weight. Cigarettes are a powerful appetite suppressant and girls get used to this effect. This suggestion seems not to cut much ice in our hospital canteen where rather plump nurses are buying polystyrene containers full of chips to go outside into the hospital grounds to smoke.

The relationship between smoking cigarettes and lung cancer is now clear. This comes from the correlation of smoking and the disease in both retrospective and prospective studies. There is a dose-dependent relationship between the amount of tobacco consumed and the incidence of cancer. The way in which the tobacco is smoked is also important. Longer cigarettes, the lack of filter-tips and complete inhaling of every puff also increase cancer incidence. Animal experiments have shown the carcinogenic potential of tobacco products. Finally, a classical epidemiological study by Sir Richard Doll among British doctors who stopped smoking in the early 1960's, demonstrated clearly that by doing so, the incidence of cancer falls to normal.

The powerful tobacco lobby has raised several objections to this apparently clear-cut evidence. Their major objection is that smokers are a group who have a different behaviour pattern with regard to food intake, life-style and environment when compared to non-smokers. The causative factors for the higher incidence of lung cancer could come from any of these features rather than directly from smoking. Such objections can now be discounted in view of the accumulated data.

Diagnosis

Lung cancer can present through symptoms arising from the primary tumour, metastatic spread or its non-metastatic complications. The commonest presenting symptoms are those caused by the primary tumour. These include cough, shortness of breath, blood-stained sputum, chest pain and persistent chest infections which recur despite several courses of antibiotics. In more than 90% of patients, the primary tumour arises in the main bronchi within 2 cm of the junction between the left and right bronchus. It causes symptoms by obstructing the bronchus, which in turn results in consolidation and collapse of the distal lung. Local invasion can also result in pleural or pericardial effusion; invasion of the chest wall can cause pain; difficulty in swallowing occurs from pressure on the oesophagus, while extension around the great veins can result in the syndrome of superior vena cava compression. The invasion of local nerves results in Horner's syndrome (sympathetic chain), hoarseness (recurrent laryngeal nerve palsy), brachial plexus syndrome or dyspnoea due to involvement of the phrenic nerve with subsequent paralysis of the diaphragm on one side.

Common sites for metastases are bone, liver and brain, although almost any organ can be infiltrated by this tumour. A group of non-metastatic complications has fascinated physicians for many years and are commonly discussed in medical examinations of doctors at all levels. Fortunately, these are relatively rare, and their mechanisms are often not fully understood.

The initial diagnosis of a patient with a possible lung cancer includes full blood count, urea and electrolytes, liver function tests, chest x-ray, CT scan and bronchoscopic biopsy. The advent of the flexible fibreoptic bronchoscope has made direct biopsy a much simpler affair which can be performed in the outpatient clinic under local anaesthetic. A biopsy is essential to plan radical therapy. A CT scan of the chest may also be useful to make sure that the disease is indeed confined to the mediastinal area. Mediastinoscopy – the passage of a tube into the mediastinum – and the biopsy of lymph nodes there, is sometimes of value in obtaining tissue if bronchoscopy fails. From these investigations, the stage of the disease can be assessed and the precise classification determined.

There are four main types of lung cancer with differing incidence rates. Non-small cell lung cancer (80%):

- squamous cell cancer
- adenocarcinoma
- large cell carcinoma
- small cell lung cancer (20%)

Squamous carcinomas arise almost exclusively in the main bronchi and spread slowly via the mediastinal lymph node chain. Adenocarcinomas may arise peripherally from the little sacs of the lung. A biopsy may be difficult to obtain on bronchoscopy, and either a lung biopsy or thoractotomy may be required to differentiate these lesions from benign granulomas. Small cell lung cancer arises from neuroectodermal cells and spreads rapidly. The majority of patients with small cell carcinoma have metastases at the time of presentation.

The lung is also a common site for metastatic spread from other tumours. The filtering effect of the pulmonary vasculature traps circulating tumour cells which grow in the well oxygenated environment. Tumours of the breast, prostate, testis and colon can all be found growing as masses inside the lung. Another pattern of secondary spread is through the lymphatics, giving rise to a fluffy appearance arising at the centre of a chest x-ray. This pattern is called lymphangitis carcinomatosa, and is most common with breast cancer but can also occur with pancreatic and other gastrointestinal primaries.

Treatment

The two most important factors in deciding the best treatment plan for an individual patient include the stage of the disease and the pathological type. In view of the different patterns of metastatic spread for small cell lung cancer and its unique sensitivity to chemotherapy, the identification of this pathological type alters the overall management.

If a biopsy reveals non-small cell cancer, and this is localized, then the best chance of obtaining a cure is to remove it surgically by removing the whole of one lung (pneumonectomy) or just one lobe (lobectomy). Neither may be possible if the tumour is central or the central lymph nodes are involved by cancer. Radical radiotherapy using a planned volume, may eradicate the disease. If the disease is extensive and surgery or radiotherapy is unlikely to be curative, then chemotherapy can be tried, but results are poor. Palliative radiotherapy can often be remarkably successful in ameliorating symptoms such as pain or coughing up blood.

The treatment approach in patients with small cell cancer is rather different, in view of its potential to spread. Tumours that appear to be localized on initial investigation are treated with a combination of local radiotherapy and chemotherapy. Small cell tumours are remarkably sensitive to the effects of chemotherapy, with up to 80% of patients responding well to relatively simple regimens. Unfortunately, the disease can return rapidly, in most cases resistant to the effects of drugs. This problem of drug resistance bedevils treatment of many tumours where chemotherapy is initially successful. Patients with extensive small cell carcinoma are treated with chemotherapy, and although tumour responses are often obtained, the overall results are disappointing.

It is important to give good supportive care for all patients with lung cancer. The overall results are poor – at 5 years only some 8% of patients presenting will be alive. Attention to alleviating distressing symptoms and the continuing care of the patient after active treatment are vital. There is considerable variation in treatment policies between different centres and even between different consultants at the same centre. For example, some believe that radical radiotherapy has no role to play in the management of this disease. Arguments against radical radiotherapy include the lack of evidence to show cures in large numbers of patients. There is little evidence that overall quality of life is better in patients who receive such treatment, but there is also no doubt that some 5–10% of patients in this way are cured of their disease.

Radical radiotherapy is planned by using a CT scan at an appropriate level as a guide. The tumour to which the radical dose is to be delivered is marked and an outline of the body constructed using a flexible ruler. Structures that the radiotherapist wishes to avoid because of their sensitivity, include normal lung and spinal cord. A three-field plan is a common approach. Treatment usually takes place daily, 5 days a week over 4–6 weeks. The major side effects of this include oesophagitis, causing difficulty in swallowing, and pneumonitis. The latter may be averted to some extent by the administration of steroids in low doses. It is the pneumonitis that effectively prevents large tumours being irradiated to a radical dose.

Chemotherapy can also be used in patients whose disease has spread. There are several new drugs available which have very good effects in reducing the amount of cancer. Unfortunately, most cancers become resistant to the drugs by changing their growth patterns. Second and third line chemotherapy with different drugs is possible but the effectiveness gradually reduces. Trying to find ways to overcome this drug resistance is a research priority.

Molecular targeted therapy has greatly advanced the field of treatment for non-small cell lung cancer (NSCLC). Gefitinib (Iressa), which was the first molecular targeted therapeutic agent against a cell surface receptor (epidermal growth factor receptor – EGFR) which is often over-expressed in lung cancer, has doubled the survival time of NSCLC patients. Lung cancer develops through the activating mutations of many driver genes including EGFR, anaplastic lymphoma kinase (ALK), ROS1, BRAF and rearranged during transfection (RET) genes. Although ALK, ROS1, and RET are rare genetic abnormalities, tyrosine kinase inhibitors (TKIs) can exert dramatic therapeutic effects. They are also given regularly as tablets and have fewer side effects than chemotherapy. In addition to anticancer drugs targeting driver genes, bevacizumab specifically binds to human vascular endothelial growth factor (VEGF) and blocks its signaling pathway. The VEGF signal blockade suppresses new blood vessel formation in tumor tissues and inhibits tumor growth. There is also immunotherapy (see Chapter 3), which is a promising approach in a variety of cancers. Antitumor immune responses are suppressed in cancer patients, and cancer cells escape from the immune surveillance mechanism. Immune checkpoint inhibitors (ICIs) are antibodies that target the primary escape mechanisms, immune checkpoints. Patients who respond to these drugs often experience long lasting benefit.

Lymphoma

These tumours arise from cells of the lymphoid system – which consists of lymph nodes that are scattered around the body but most easily felt in the neck – connected by a tiny series of pipes called lymphatics. Lymphomas make up only 4% of all human cancers so are relatively rare. Some are easy to cure, while others may be responsive in the short term to both radiotherapy and chemotherapy but recur frequently eventually. The classification of lymphomas has bedeviled medical students, physicians and pathologists for the last three decades. More recently, the confusion has been heightened by the availability of monoclonal antibodies – magic bullets – which can accurately classify different sub-populations of normal and malignant lymphocytes. Antibodies such as rituximab can be used to treat certain lymphomas.

There are two types of malignant lymphoma. The first, Hodgkin Lymphoma (previously known as Hodgkin's Disease), is relatively well characterized pathologically and the treatment strategy is well worked out. Non-Hodgkin Lymphomas, on the other hand, represent an area of considerable confusion, both to the pathologist and clinician. The vocabulary is very confusing to everybody. You wouldn't expect a supermarket fruit shelf to have apples on one shelf and then call all the other fruits non apples and leave you the customer to sort through them. But that's just what we clinicians do.

Hodgkin Lymphoma

The neoplasm arising from lymph nodes was first described by a Guy's Hospital physician in London, Thomas Hodgkin, in 1832. It characteristically presents in a young patient with lymph node swelling often in the neck area, which is non-tender, mobile and noted by the patient incidentally. Symptoms can occur. These include fever, weight loss, sweats at night (which may be drenching at times requiring a change of night clothes), generalised itchiness and a curious syndrome of alcohol induced pain in the area of the disease. Occasionally, it is the latter which draws attention to the lymph node swelling. Other symptoms may develop if specific organs are invaded.

Diagnosis

The first task for the doctor seeing a patient with a possible lymphoma of whatever type is to make a precise histological diagnosis by biopsy. Needle biopsies are unlikely to produce samples in which the architectural pattern can be recognized. Special stains are used to precisely identify the origin of the abnormal cells. For this reason, the excision of a whole lymph node under general anaesthesia, if necessary, is preferred so enough tissue can be examined. If lymphoma is found the full extent of the disease is assessed by staging investigations.

The combination of history, physical examination and investigations allows a precise clinical staging to be made of the disease in an individual patient. In 1971, a group of physicians met in Ann Arbor, USA, to establish the most useful way in which to classify the stage. Their system is now widely used and is of great relevance to the choice of treatment and the comparison of results from different centres.

In addition to the location of the disease, the presence of symptoms is also used to help stage the patient. Only three symptoms have been found to be of prognostic value. These are weight loss, fever, night sweats. The letter A is used to designate patients without symptoms and B for those with two or more symptoms known to affect prognosis. The staging classification is based on prognostic data collected by several groups over many years. There is a clear progression in terms of prognosis between patients with stage I disease through to stage IV; using this system the precise extent of the disease in a patient can be simply stated. For example, a patient with stage IIIsB disease has involvement of lymph nodes on both sides of the diaphragm together with the spleen and has two of the three B symptoms.

A problem that arose in the early 1970s, when effective chemotherapy started being widely used, was the difficulty in accurately staging abdominal disease. A group of patients could be identified who had involvement of the spleen or lymph nodes at the back of the abdomen detectable only by laparotomy. For this reason, a staging laparotomy – an operation to open the abdomen purely for diagnostic purposes – became a common procedure in those about to be treated with local radiotherapy alone. The advent of CT and MRI scanning and the better definition of prognostic groups within patients of the same stage have resulted in an almost total decline of this major surgical undertaking.

Radiotherapy

The best treatment for Hodgkin's disease is still local radiotherapy, provided that this can totally encompass all sites of tumour. This is always the case in stage I and usually in stage II. Indeed, there are some who advocate radiotherapy using irradiation of the total lymph node system for patients with stage III disease as well. For stage IV with bone marrow or organ infiltration, chemotherapy is necessary. In patients treated with local radiotherapy the precise extent of the disease, must be determined if a geographical miss is to be avoided. A dose of 40Gy in 20 treatments over a 4-week period is usually given a much lower dose than given to cure many other cancers. As most patients present with neck nodes, often with axillary involvement, a technique which involves the cutting of lead blocks to shield the lung is often used. This allows the mediastinum, neck and both axillae to be irradiated in one continuous field. The pattern of light beam on the patient while setting up such treatment resembles a mantle and hence it is called mantle radiotherapy.

Chemotherapy

For patients with stage IIIB or IV disease chemotherapy is front line therapy. Many single agents have been used in the past for the treatment of this condition, but remissions were usually of short duration. In 1965 a combination of four drugs – nitrogen mustard, vincristine, procarbazine and prednisone (MOPP) – was discovered to be particularly effective in bringing about a high rate of cure and heralded a new era of combination therapy. Most physicians now replace MOPP with more effective and less unpleasant combinations such as ABVD (adriamycin, bleomycin, vincristine and dacarbazine). Four courses of this regimen are given, and the patient is then reinvestigated. If there is complete remission, a further two cycles are given, and the patient followed up at regular intervals. If, on the other hand, resolution of disease is slow, then two cycles beyond that required to achieve complete remission are given.

The overall cure rate of patients with Hodgkin's disease is extremely high, but still dependent to some extent on the stage of the disease. Thus, stage I patients have a 95% chance of being alive and disease free 5 years after treatment, while those with stage IV who are treated with chemotherapy have an 80% chance. Patients whose disease recurs can still be treated successfully and cured. Those that are treated first with radiotherapy can be given chemotherapy, while those who have already received chemotherapy can receive alternative regimens.

Factors affecting the prognosis in addition to stage include the histological type, nodular sclerosis and lymphocyte predominant are more favourable than the rare mixed cellularity or lymphocyte depleted type; age, young patients fare better than old; and sex, females have a better prognosis than males. Hodgkin Lymphoma disease is a good example of a tumour whose cure rate has improved dramatically over the last three decades.

Non-Hodgkin Lymphoma
This is an extremely heterogeneous group of diseases, for which the classification still remains in dispute. The problem is that 20 years ago pathologists had no access to the lymphocyte typing reagents now available. Their classification was based solely on the appearance of the abnormal cells down the microscope and the staining patterns with chemicals. The first reproducible system to be used was that devised by Frank Rappaport, a Californian pathologist. It was then widely adapted and modified by many investigators. By 1970 no-one could call themselves an expert in the pathology of lymphoma unless he had formulated his own system. The plethora of classification systems led to total confusion, and in some cases, incorrect diagnostic labels were attached.

To the clinician, however, there are basically two patterns of disease. The first carries a good prognosis. It is represented by the nodular lymphomas, and these are of B-cell origin. They respond well to radiotherapy or to simple chemotherapy with oral alkylating agents such as chlorambucil. Although a high incidence of complete tumour regression is obtained, when the disease is widespread, recurrences often occur.

The second group runs a much more aggressive clinical course and is typified by the diffuse lymphocytic lymphomas. This group responds well to both chemotherapy and radiotherapy, but unfortunately relapses, often with widespread systemic disease, such as bone marrow involvement, so causing multisystem failure.

The investigative approach to these patients is like those with Hodgkin Lymphoma. A biopsy is essential to make an accurate diagnosis, and this is followed by the same staging procedures described above. Patients with lymphoma of good prognosis are treated with local radiotherapy or simple oral anti-cancer drugs such as chlorambucil, depending on stage. Aggressive combination chemotherapy such as the R-CHOP combination (rituximab, cyclophosphamide, doxorubicin, vincristine and prednisolone) is reserved for those patients with widespread poor prognostic histology. Extremely aggressive chemotherapy with the administration of normally supra-lethal doses of drugs followed by bone marrow rescue, has been attempted with moderate success. It seems that dose escalation alone is inadequate to prevent the development of drug resistance that eventually supervenes. More recently a variety of new drugs have had shown significant benefit. The overall outlook for patients with Non Hodgkin Lymphoma is excellent with the majority surviving 5 years.

CAR-T cell therapy is a type of treatment that uses normal T lymphocytes from the patient's own immune system to destroy their lymphoma. They are modified in the laboratory to produce Chimeric Antigen Receptor T cells. T cells are a type of white blood cell. T cells usually recognise and kill abnormal cancer cells. However, cancer cells are good at tricking T cells, either by looking very similar to healthy cells or by sending signals that tell the T cells not to attack them.

In CAR-T cell therapy, T cells are collected and sent off to a lab. In the lab, they are genetically modified so they can recognise and stick to a particular protein on the surface of your lymphoma cells. These genetically modified T cells are known as CAR-T cells. It's early days to fully understand the role of this treatment. It's very expensive mainly because it is so individualised. The costs are often over £500,000 per patient. Studies in cancers other than lymphoma have not shown much promise probably because the strength of the molecular flags that can be recognised by the immune system are relatively weak.

Head and neck cancer

Cancers of the head and neck refer to those arising from the upper respiratory tract and the food passages. Brain tumours and those of the eye are excluded from this group of cancers. They tend to occur in people over seventy although it is possible but rare for young people to develop a head and neck cancer. The patients are predominantly male with a three to one ratio between the incidence in men and women.

The causes of head and neck cancer include smoking, drinking strong spirits, poor dental hygiene, infection with the wart virus or human papilloma virus and dietary factors. However, in most patients no single factor can be identified as causative.

Tumours are classified by the site in which they arise. This can be the lip or the cavity of the back of the nose (nasopharynx), voice box (larynx) or the pharynx which is the bit from the back of the tongue where the windpipe (trachea) and gullet (oesophagus) split off. In the trachea the tumours become lung cancer and, in the oesophagus, oesophageal cancer.

The treatment offered depends on how far the tumour has spread and its type as examined down a microscope in the pathology laboratory. Some types of head and neck cancer have an excellent outcome. Cancer of the larynx arises in the vocal cords and spreads only very slowly to the lymph nodes in the neck and then onwards to the rest of the body. Because it affects speech by resulting in hoarseness as a very early symptom, it is picked up early and so most patients are cured by radiotherapy. On the other hand, tumours of the pharynx, especially in older people, are slow to be picked up and often spread into the lymph nodes prior to diagnosis. For this reason, the outcome is much poorer.

Treatments offered to patients with head and neck cancer follow a common pattern. They include all three of the major modalities of cancer treatment; surgery, radiotherapy and chemotherapy. The order in which things are done depends on the exact clinical circumstance in a patient. For this reason, head and neck cancer is complicated by a near individualisation of treatment strategies. This is usually decided on by a multidisciplinary team consisting of specialist surgeons, oncologists, radiotherapists, dental surgeons and reconstructive and plastic surgeons.

When a patient is suspected of having a head and neck cancer they are first referred to an ENT clinic (ear, nose and throat). Here mirrors are used to visualise as far as possible the area behind the tongue and at the back of the nose. This can be uncomfortable and so usually a bit of local anaesthetic is sprayed onto the very sensitive mucosa that lines the air passages. Doctors soon get quite expert at doing it quickly and with as little discomfort as possible. To take a biopsy it is usual to examine patients under an anaesthetic, usually as a day case. The patient is put to sleep and then a small piece of the abnormal area that has been visualised is removed for pathology review.

Most cancers of the head and neck are squamous tumours arising from the cells that make the epithelium of the passages. Other types of cancers also arise and may well be treated slightly differently. These include adenocarcinomas from glandular tissue and lymphomas from lymphatic tissue. As well as a biopsy some form of imaging is used to exactly work out where the cancer is as part of the staging process. The usual technologies are MRI or CT scanning to give very good views of all the structures in the region and really allow the multidisciplinary team to make an informed decision about what to do for an individual patient.

Surgery
Surgery is the usual first line of treatment for most cancers except those that have spread widely or those that arise in the larynx. If the tumour has spread widely then it is unlikely that surgery could be helpful without some form of remarkable reconstruction of this very sensitive area. Surgery is not the primary treatment of laryngeal cancer as radiotherapy is so effective at giving a good result in terms of cure from cancer and at the same time preserving the integrity of the voice box.

Surgery requires several days in hospital, and it may be recommended to remove not just the primary tumour but also the lymph nodes on the same side of the neck. This is called a radical neck dissection. The aim of this is to remove all the cancer that may have spread into the lymph nodes. In someone with a very high risk of disease spreading it may be done with no imaging evidence of lymph node involvement. Again the lymph nodes are sent to the pathologist for his opinion about whether the nodes are involved or not.

Radiotherapy
Modern radiotherapy has transformed the treatment of head and neck cancer by using the latest technologies of intensity modulated radiotherapy (IMRT) and image guided radiotherapy (IGRT) at very precise dose distributions exactly around the cancer and its likely sites of spread can be obtained with minimal damage to normal tissue. This is vital in this area as the mucosa is very sensitive to damage caused by radiotherapy. Treatment is usually given over a long period of time; often thirty treatments over six weeks. It is also important that the patient is immobilised during treatment to make sure the delivery is as precise as possible. This is usually done by constructing an individual face mask which is used to fix the patient to the couch. It sounds uncomfortable but really is not at all unpleasant. I have had one made for me; it is rather like going to Madame Tussauds, I imagine.

During the first two weeks there are usually no side effects. They begin in the third week with some irritation and perhaps even some ulceration at the back of the mouth and in the throat. This can be very uncomfortable.

There are a whole range of medications that will prevent some of this discomfort, from simple mouth washes to antibiotic cover if infection occurs. The side effects of radiotherapy continue for two weeks after the treatment stops as normal cells find it difficult to repair any damage after radiotherapy.

Eating bland foods and avoiding alcohol and smoking are essential during and after radiotherapy. Some patients lose a lot of weight during treatment. They can be helped enormously by a dietician who will make recommendations for well tolerated high calorie supplements which can be obtained from chemists or health food shops. Radiotherapy also has long term side effects, but these are now much lower in occurrence because of better targeting with sophisticated planning and delivery equipment.

Proton beam therapy may have advantages for some patients although this is not currently easily available in the UK. It has the advantage of reducing damage to the many critical structures in that lie right next to the cancer.

Chemotherapy

There are two reasons to use chemotherapy in head and neck cancer. The first is called adjuvant or neoadjuvant treatment and it is given either before or after surgery and radiotherapy. Giving chemotherapy before other treatment modalities may be useful to shrink a tumour that has spread locally to include areas that would leave lasting damage if surgically excised. It may also be given after surgery if it is thought the risk of recurrence is very high. So, for example, if a patient has known lymph node involvement in the neck, the surgeon may remove the nodes but it is highly likely even after a radical neck dissection some small areas of cancer may be left behind. The aim of adjuvant chemotherapy is to mop these tumour cells up so that they do not grow back. Sometimes chemotherapy is given in a timed way with radiotherapy. This is because it can enhance the damage radiation causes to cancer cells without increasing the side effects of treatment. This is called chemo-radiotherapy.

Chemotherapy is also used for patients with metastatic cancer where the cancer has spread to other sites. This often includes other lymph nodes groups such as those as the other side of the neck to the main cancer and to the axilla. Head and neck cancers can also spread to the lung, liver or indeed any organ of the body. Drugs used for treatment of metastatic cancer are the same as those used before in the adjuvant setting. These include Cisplatin, Carboplatin, Taxol, Gemcitabine, Capecitabine, Cetuximab and 5 Fluorouracil.

Exactly how the chemotherapy is given varies from centre to centre. In some it means coming to a Day Ward every three weeks for a two-to-three-hour infusion. Other centres use small portable pumps to give one of the drugs, the 5 Fluorouracil for five days and every three weeks the other drugs. There is a lot of discussion about the best way to do things and no clear answers. This results in the variation.

There have been dramatic improvements in the overall outcome in the treatment of these relatively rare types of cancer. It is a classic example where a complete team is necessary and not just doctors. Important members of the team are dieticians, speech therapists, specialist nurses and counsellors. If you or someone you care for has head and neck cancer the most important thing is to go to a unit that has the necessary team in place to help you. Going private to a single clinician is not going to get you the best care.

Chapter Nine: Complementary and alternative medicine

Use wisely as an adjunct to conventional therapy but beware of unscrupulous quacks

Over ten million people in the world are diagnosed as having cancer each year. For many it will be the first time they face a life-threatening disease with a high level of uncertainty in terms of outcome. Complementary medicine interventions of many types have become increasingly popular with patients. Surveys have shown repeatedly that up to 60% of women and 30% of men with cancer are taking some form of complementary or alternative therapy in the UK. Some of these are simple and cheap – a limited number of weekly group therapy sessions whilst others, involving prolonged one to one professional contact, are more costly and realistically can only be used selectively. Practitioners often work in isolation and provide just a single modality or type of treatment, rather than a holistic service. There are many options available but very little true integration around the needs of an individual person living with cancer.

Supportive therapies
There is very little research in this area and most of the published academic literature is anecdotal. A further problem is the multiplicity of treatments often given by dedicated but single modality practitioners. In 1982 the Bristol Cancer Help Centre (now Penny Brohn Cancer Care), was founded to pioneer the use of a whole range of complementary therapies for cancer. The initial approach was to provide an alternative to conventional care but over the last two decades the centre has moved to a truly integrative approach. This has spawned out into various conventional cancer centres in both the NHS and private sectors. Two leading groups are at Hammersmith Hospital, now part of Imperial College, and the Harley Street Clinic.

In both centres an integrated approach with 6 sessions of therapy offered as part of routine radiotherapy or chemotherapy. The aim of these hospital-based programmes is to give the patient psychological and physical support during a time of potential great stress. This may allow patients to withstand some of the toxicities of conventional therapy so enhancing their chances of survival. Complementary medicine here is not used as an alternative to conventional medical care.

Simple low-cost strategies are currently prominent. These include counselling in which the patient's hidden fears and anxieties are explored more fully – not in the context of the disease – but in the context of a whole person. Modern cancer treatment is essentially mechanistic and a more whole person centred approach helps many people. Cancer support groups have been around for many years. Even in waiting areas patients share their fears and anxieties and get relief from doing so. A properly run patient support group with a professional counsellor is of great help. Clearly patients have to be willing to go. A good facilitator avoids repeated discussion of specific individual symptoms and encourages the less vocal members of the group to participate fully in the discussion.

Treatment with radiotherapy and chemotherapy is not always pleasant and there is the additional worry that the disease will not be cured or that palliation will only be obtained with considerable side effects. Relaxation in a quiet room with an experienced therapist enables patients to get through their treatment more easily. The visualisation of healing images is also helpful to many patients who can see radiation and drugs as a powerful, destructive force to their tumours.

Modern medicine often uses the military metaphor where we wage war on a disease such as cancer destroying it with magic bullets, guided missiles, targeted drugs and try to avoid collateral damage. Whilst such metaphors may be helpful to patients, getting to a level of acceptance of the situation and healing is far more challenging. Integrated medicine can help with this. A boutique approach of complementary therapy is used for cancer: counselling, acupuncture, homeopathy, herbalism, naturopathy, meditation, visualization, relaxation, reflexology, massage, osteopathy, hypnotherapy and nutritional support.

Surprisingly, certain complementary therapies are already covered within the NHS. There is no evidence that homeopathy is of more value in cancer treatment than other complementary therapies, yet several outlets exist for a free homeopathic consultation and treatment in the NHS. There needs to be a rethinking of funding to a more balanced format allowing other modalities to be offered side by side with orthodox care. The cost of providing psychosocial support is only a fraction of that used for cancer treatments, many of which are still given in situations where they have little benefit. Diverting resources to supportive care could provide a new paradigm in modern healthcare.

Those involved in delivering the softer side of cancer care tend not to be very hard-nosed about business issues, but health economics is becoming an increasingly used policy tool in rich and poor healthcare environments alike. Although we may sometimes find it uncomfortable, we ration medical care delivery all the time often without realising it. Economic analysis allows us to do the job better without imposing our own prejudices, values and baggage.

Achieving integrated care

Understanding the costs and benefits of integrated medicine requires three inputs. Firstly, what is the delivery cost involved? 90% of this is for professional salaries, easy to determine within a defined environment. The second issue is how much benefit in terms of quality-of-life gain does it actually deliver? Measuring quality of life is not an exact science but reasonably reliable instruments are out there. Some believers and indeed a few randomised controlled trials, already suggest that simple psychological interventions can bring about a modest survival improvement in cancer patients, but the studies have been mostly inadequately powered for the purposes of economics. The third and perhaps most difficult factor to assess accurately is how much money does effective intervention save the medical care system, the patient and society.

Medical care forms only part of the overall financial equation. Indirect cancer related costs to the patient include loss of earnings, travel and accommodation and the need for carers to take time off their work. These are far more difficult costs to estimate and vary enormously by socio-economic grouping. Can good psycho-social care get people back to work faster and more effectively? Probably so, but what does this really mean financially? The price tag for society in supporting distressed, depressed and in some cases disturbed cancer patients is impossible to assess. Marital breakdown, family disintegration and mental illness in carers can all be part of this price. Of course, the potential for financial saving goes into many different pockets and so estimating the reduction in overall medical care costs is a good place to start for future research.

The rise in the popularity of complementary and alternative medicines for cancer reflects in part the inability of orthodox medicine to deliver what people want – hope in a caring environment and the increased ability to cope with the stress caused by the disease. The internet now lists over a billion cancer sites. Agency relationships in which healthcare professionals act as the patient's agent making decisions on complex technical matters such as the benefits of different types of adjuvant chemotherapy have increasingly put the patient more fully in the driving seat. Different people respond differently to these approaches. Some find the information bewildering and are not able to assimilate the options. Others get confused and frightened and are pushed further into denial. However, good integrated medicine is rapidly becoming an essential tool in cancer care as the technical options increase and the patient plays a greater role in their choice of their own treatment.

If you feel you would like to explore other methods of treatment in addition to those offered conventionally, you should voice your needs and ask about the complementary medicine facilities available within the hospital itself, within the locality and on a national basis. The response you obtain is likely to vary enormously between different doctors and nurses. The medical profession is now more receptive to this approach and fully aware that different patients have differing needs and wishes.

Counselling in the hospital setting is becoming more widely available and in this respect, complementary medicine may well support patients as a helpful way of coming to terms with the diagnosis and coping with conventional treatment. Indeed caring for cancer patients carries its own stress and staff may actually benefit from the availability of regular counselling themselves. Discussing difficult or upsetting problems relating to patients often helps to ease the burden. No two patients react in the same way to the diagnosis so their approach to treatment and ability to carry on with their lives afterwards will also differ. Some want to abdicate responsibility to their specialist, others want to feel completely in control and therefore need as much information about their disease and its treatment as possible. Some have fixed ideas about their illness and its likely outcome, which no amount of persuasion can dislodge. Just as everyone will have a different approach to their illness, the help and information provided must be tailored to meet their individual requirements.

The extreme alternatives

We recognize that a proportion of doctors are very cynical about the use of complementary medicine but by the same token some alternative practitioners pour scorn on conventional treatment. Both extremes are unhelpful for patient and doctor alike. They may serve to undermine your confidence in the treatment you have had or likely to be offered in the future or compromise your relationship with the doctor offering conventional therapy if you bring in the baggage from a negative complementary therapist with you.

Provided one form of treatment does not compromise the effectiveness of the other it is best to be open-minded and receptive to both groups. For example, a patient receiving abdominal radiotherapy may insist on religiously adhering to a strict vegan diet. The high intake of largely raw food contains much roughage and is likely to stimulate the bowel making the side effects of radiotherapy much worse. The best way to handle the tension inevitably existing between the complementary and orthodox world is to be honest with both parties and choose a route that you feel most comfortable with. Most doctors are fine with simple techniques such as counseling, relaxation, reflexology, meditation, yoga, visualization, healing, acupuncture and hypnotherapy.

Things get more difficult when alternative therapies are given that mimic conventional treatments that are not registered with the drug authorities. Homeopathy is perhaps one of the most difficult areas and herbal remedies, extreme nutritional therapies, psychic surgery and apparent wonder cures are all frowned on by most oncologists, simply because they haven't produced the sort of evidence that allow these techniques to be used widely and some are extremely expensive as much as modern chemotherapy. When a cult grows up about one specific treatment delivered in clinics internationally, people travel enormous distances and pay huge amounts of money to get what they think is the best treatment for them. Over the last decade there have been all sorts of extreme claims for cure from substances as diverse as apricot pips, shark's cartilage, curcumin, coffee enemas, extreme diets and cannabis oil. None have stood the test of a clinical trial and the accounts purporting to be studies are really just anecdotes.

There are also the conspiracy theories that doctors, and the pharmaceutical industry are in cahoots with each other and hide relatively simple cures for cancer that are cheap and not patentable. For several years I was heckled by a very charming elderly gentleman who had once been a scientist and believed that promethazine, a tranquillizer, was the cure for cancer. He wrote me letters, attended my lectures, and poured scorn on all orthodox cancer treatment. His solution was just to give everyone promethazine, an old drug that has long lost its patent. I tried to rationalize with him, but he was having none of it. Several of my colleagues had the same problem. If there really was an effective simple anti-cancer drug out there, we would use it whatever its provenance. There is no bias against it, it's just that we need to see the evidence.

Chapter Ten: The politics of cancer

How to find out what you can get and then get it

There is a great deal of good, published guidance on the care available in the NHS. This tells you what you can get and how to get it. The best set of cancer treatment guidelines in the world come from the US and are those of the National Comprehensive Cancer Network and can be found in detail at www.nccn.org. This represents a synthesis of good practice from the top 32 cancer centres in America. It's a brilliant tool for oncologists but you can access it too.

Go to this site and log in as a health professional. It will give you gold plated care pathways for every type of cancer except the rarest. The recommended diagnostics – scans, blood tests and pathology are listed. The broad sequence of treatments – surgery, radiotherapy, chemotherapy – are all in there. Contrast the contents to the much less detailed and less rigorous UK sites such as those of the NHS, Macmillan or Cancer Research UK. The NHS site especially is heavily patronizing and assumes you are plain stupid.

Research the strengths and weaknesses of your own health system. Every physician, provider or insurer has their own set of rules and guidelines, just like any organisation. The costs of cancer treatment come in many parts – diagnosis, surgery, radiotherapy, chemotherapy, drugs and follow up tests and visits. You may well need several or indeed all of those. The cost pressures will come at different points in the process depending on your healthcare system. Some are generous with surgery but restrict access to the super-expensive drugs. With others, it will be the other way. There is enormous variation on what is offered to patients even in a national system such as the NHS and it changes with time. Post code prescribing of high-cost drugs and technology has been with us since the birth of the NHS in 1948.

You need to make yourself aware of where the cost pressures are. That way you can start to work out how you can make sure they are not applied to you. You need to make sure you really are seeking something that others are getting for the same type of cancer. Check all possible sources – your doctors, specialist nurses, other patients, cancer help lines. If you feel you are missing out, make a fuss – politely. In Britain's

NHS for example, and despite what many people think, you can get first-class cancer treatment. It will be as good as anything in the world. The trouble is it may not all be available in the same place.

Some hospitals will offer excellent treatment in one class of cancer, but not in others. Just across the county borders it will be the other way around. Some offer a complete range of drugs – others will have huge restrictions. You don't want to end up getting second-best treatment when the first-class healthcare is available just a few miles away and at no extra cost. Fortunately, whilst care varies, your rights do not. You're entitled to the best care anywhere. But again, you won't necessarily be offered it. You'll need to find out where the best is and then make sure you get it. We will first look at how high-cost cancer drugs are rationed and then the very variable access to precision radiotherapy.

Let me give you a bit of insight into what is going on in the UK around cancer drug access, as it a very good example of politicians trying to deceive the public though a very complex set of policies. It goes on everywhere from Obamacare in the US, the French mandatory social insurance plans, and even the Chinese public health system. Survey after survey has shown that health is the most important election issue for the floating voter. Taxes, education, roads and immigration are all big issues but health and particularly the NHS is the biggest issue to most. And in health what is the most important disease? 72% of participants in a large survey said cancer. No surprise then that no politician anywhere wants to be seen rationing cancer drugs. So how are our current lot distancing themselves from the problem?

British cancer drug politics have moved on considerably over the last few years in an attempt to avoid the need for politically unpopular top-up payments in the NHS whereby patients have to pay separately out of their own pocket for high cost cancer drugs. Since April 2011 until now a much heralded £200m a year Cancer Drugs Fund has been created so that the Conservative Party election manifesto could be delivered.

"We are strengthening the National Institute of Clinical Excellence (NICE) and have already created the £200 million per year Cancer Drugs Fund, so that all patients can get access to the drugs and treatments their doctors think they need." – David Cameron 2010.

Implementing this rather inconsistent policy in the last two years has resulted in major changes in how high-cost cancer drugs are funded. NICE is supposed to judge whether a drug is worth the money by valuing a year of your life at around £30,000. If an intervention costs above this it is not recommended for NHS use. Of course, it's riddled with inconsistencies. Children with rare enzyme deficiencies are regularly given drugs that cost over £150,000 a year to keep them alive. Do you think we should stop this and just let them die? An attempt in Birmingham several years ago failed.

Most UK oncologists are only just beginning to realize that what's now happening in cancer is actually political fudging. The real problem is an increase in inequity in what is supposedly a national service. Post code prescribing is rife. The drugs you can get depend on who's making the decision for you. There is now good evidence that better educated middle class patients are accessing cancer drugs more easily because of the complexity of the bureaucracy surrounding their acquisition. Why, because they are playing the system better. You must do the same. Use the websites referred to in the appendix to give you detailed guidance.

There are five processes in place – all controlled by government agencies. A man from Mars would find the complexity unbelievable! It's designed that way.

1. The National Institute for Health and Care Excellence (NICE) makes recommendations that determine whether a treatment will be reimbursed by the NHS. The drugs are bought by provider hospitals and reimbursed by the 230 local Clinical Commissioning Groups (CCGs). If NICE has not approved or rejected a drug it can then be requested through the Cancer Drugs Fund. This avoids the need for politicians to look as though they are rationing drugs, which of course they are.

2. Until 2012 the Cancer Drug Fund of £200m was administered by the 13 Strategic Health Authorities in England. These were disbanded and replaced by NHS England. Most of the staff got made redundant at great expense to you the taxpayer and were then hired again by a different agency within the NHS. No machinery was in place to cover the transition of this fund to CCGs as the Drug Fund was supposed to end in April 2014.

3. The big idea was that we would wake up on the morning of April 1st 2014 with a brilliant new Value Based Pricing (VBP) scheme – the better the value of the drug in terms of patient benefit – judged by length and quality of life – the more the NHS would be prepared to pay for it. That would seem a perfectly reasonable

solution. A General Election loomed, and nobody really told the pharmaceutical industry how it was all going to work. Predictably it never happened as Big Pharma simply refused to play ball and so we all muddled through with an expanded version of the Drugs Fund, currently at £400m a year and a complex patient access scheme. It all is supposed to end just as this book goes to press. But dear reader, don't hold your breath – I predict there will be more obfuscation and muddling through.

4. The patient access schemes (PAS) created by industry starting in 2007 specifically for the NHS to appease UK politicians. As the table below shows this contains a variety of schemes which have much in common with retail markets. This is not surprising as they were devised by retailers hired by the drug industry. All have had to be agreed in advance with PASLU – the PAS Liaison Unit in the DH – a bunch of jobsworths in a rather tacky office in Holborn in London.

   Some examples of access scheme cancer drugs are given below. All drugs have two names the generic name (no capitals) and the trade name (capital). The trade name is chosen by the manufacturer and is glitzy, positive and easy to pronounce. The names are made up by brainstorming by very bright twenty-somethings in the advertising and marketing world. Drug companies pay several million dollars to come up with a good name.

   Nobody currently has any idea how Value Based Pricing will work for cancer. I suspect it will be quietly forgotten about and we'll go back to NICE and a national prescribing list with some sort of exceptional case system. You can of course always become exceptional by going privately and simply buying the drug.

5. A new scheme without a name as yet to get new medicines into the clinic in the UK as fast as possible where they are used to treat life threatening diseases such as cancer. It was announced with great fanfare. I bet it will be called the Innovative Medicines Access Scheme or something like it – IMAS for short. The deal is this. If a company has a drug that's not yet licensed it can sell it if the purchasing body in the NHS is willing to buy it for a patient. The scheme is very short on detail about who calls the shots on this and even shorter on where the money is going to come from. It's going to be a real headache to administer and to avoid yet more inequity.

To get a drug the patient's consultant must fill in a load of forms, give them to the hospital pharmacy who cost the treatment and send it on for approval. The numbers that pass vary enormously around the country hence the post code lottery.

As you can imagine the current situation with a predominantly PAS-driven new market is producing an intolerable administrative burden on NHS providers and is not sustainable. At Hammersmith Hospital we estimate that only 30% of possible PAS reimbursement money is currently actually collected by the hospital. There is simply no real incentive as the costs are just passed to the CCGs [Clinical Commissioning Groups] who are usually unaware of these schemes.

So, it's all one big headache for all of us. What can you do to get the best for yourself? As I have found the key is to make sure you really are seeking something that others are getting for the same type of cancer. Check with all sources possible – your doctors, specialist nurses, the receptionist, other patients you meet and cancer charity telephone information services. And if you're told its not available to you, then make a big fuss.

Do not be rude. Do not shout at anyone. Don't write aggressive letters or send unpleasant threatening emails. Don't threaten to write to your MP – he couldn't care less about your health unless he can get into the local paper looking good – and above all don't lose your temper. Don't go to a lawyer and don't send a formal complaint about your doctors. That sort of behaviour will see doors slammed firmly shut in your face. Get your facts correct and discuss the situation calmly with your consultant. Find out if he or she agrees you are suitable and then go through the process recommended by them. They've got to be kept on your side.

You have one big advantage. As we saw earlier, your healthcare system – whether state-funded or private – will never want to admit that it is rationing the treatment potentially available to you. They are all engaged in a conspiracy to pretend that everyone they cover is getting the best healthcare possible. Simply letting the people in charge of your treatment know that you are aware of the cost pressures, and you know about all the potential treatments you could be offered, will put you an advantage. Make sure you make your point in a respectful but forceful way and they will know that they cannot fob you off with sub-standard, second-class care.

All of this is of course very British. Indeed, there are different systems in Scotland, Wales and Northern Ireland which are supposedly part of the same NHS. But wherever you are in the world the principles are the same. You can be sure political fudging is going on. You need to understand the system and play it to your advantage.

Wherever you are in the world the rationing problems are the same. Just take a look at www.genentechaccesssolutions.com. It's a site sponsored by Genentech, part of the drug giant Roche who make a few very expensive cancer drugs to combat the 'denial' letter issued by US medical insurers. It gives examples of the sort of letter you and sometimes your doctor needs to write. Of course, the language and style is very American. But the same format – rational, coherent, and concise works – in every system in any language. Use Google Translate to help if necessary.

Getting precision radiotherapy

Radiotherapy gets a lot less attention than cancer drugs in the media. This is because it's such a mystery for journalists who are nearly all Arts graduates. In Chapter Four you saw how radiotherapy has become far more precise with better targeting of cancer without significant damage to surrounding normal tissue.

Let's say you have been diagnosed with prostate cancer. After diagnosis and staging radical radiotherapy (that means the aim is cure) has been recommended and you agree. There are currently 73 places you can go for treatment in Britain – 58 in the NHS and 15 in the private sector. To make matters more complex a significant number of NHS patients are treated in private centres under contract. These contracts are short term and may be cancer type and post code specific – so they are very difficult to negotiate at an individual patient level.

Your research has rightly shown that you would benefit in terms of long-term results by being given the latest form of precision radiotherapy using IMRT (Intensity Modulated Radiotherapy) and daily image guidance (IGRT). Yet if we look at the current data returns on availability to NHS England it is clear there is huge variability of the availability of this technology around the country. Even more scandalous, nearly all centres are fully equipped to deliver both IMRT and IGRT but yet many have not yet started using their equipment.

Drugs are relatively simple – you either get what you want or you don't. But with radiotherapy you have to be treated at one centre so you need to know that the centre nearest to you and so the most convenient place to be treated is up to scratch. If it's not then get a referral to somewhere else. I'm always amazed how rarely this actually happens. There are two ways to find out.

Firstly, ask your consultant oncologist at your visit and again before you sign the consent form if you are getting IMRT and daily IGRT.

Secondly, check on http://www.canceruk.net/about/ what radiotherapy quality factors are for your local centre. NATCANSAT (National Clinical Analysis and Specialised Applications Team) is based at Clatterbridge Hospital near Liverpool is responsible for collecting and analysing the quality and access to radiotherapy up and down the country. The situation changes by the month. The only way to judge the quality is to look at updated data. The variation is currently extreme (IMRT 2% – 100%; IGRT 3% – 100%) and there is little sign that it will improve over the next two years as all parts of the NHS are bust. If cancer centres were private companies most would be declared bankrupt – no capital reserves, inadequate earnings to pay their staff in full and a burgeoning bureaucracy of non-productive inspections, targets, returns and reports. You, the customer, are not a priority to the management. Indeed, they rather hope you will go somewhere else.

And thirdly when you go for your planning scan – a CT or MRI carried out to construct your personalised plan – ask the planning radiographers. Knowledge is power and by showing you understand the benefits of IMRT and IGRT will help you achieve your aims.

As I said at the start, the most important person is you – so you must be satisfied that you are getting the best treatment possible. Do not be put off by bureaucracy or complexity – you only get one bite at the cherry – you need to get the best type of radiotherapy from the start. Negotiate calmly without aggression and usually locked doors will simply open and a mutually satisfactory solution found.

That's why you need this book – because the later chapters will give you an insiders' guide to making sure you get the best treatment possible, regardless of cost. The next chapter gives you a summary of what cancer is and how it's treated. Obviously, it's not tailored to your problem or your country but it will help you go to the web and find out more about exactly your problem. The internet if used correctly will act as your guide to the best treatment for you that's possible today.

Chapter Eleven: Do you really want to know?

You need to take control of your situation, and understand the options and decisions

Over the years, I have told many, many people they have cancer. It is never easy, and it is never something you get used to, but as a physician it is a task with which you must become familiar. There are as many ways of taking the news as there are people. As a physician you can never really predict what precisely the reaction will be. On the surface, someone may seem optimistic, resilient and cheerful, but you have no way of knowing what they are really like. By contrast, some patients may appear weak, indecisive, morose even, when you first meet them. But faced with the appalling challenge of a life-threatening disease, they often turn out to have the strength of an oak tree.

The truth is, none of us really know how we might react until it happens to us, or to someone close to us.

You can be angry, confused, bewildered, hysterical, or simply go into denial.

But the most important thing you can do is to start to get organised, and start working out how to get the best treatment possible. The ability to cope with extreme circumstances is one of the strongest characteristics of the human race. We read the stories of the trenches in World War One, and we wonder how the men ever held themselves together under such terrible conditions, but of course most of them did. Cancer is not as bad as that. Most people will be able to get through it, even if they may not think they can at first.

In the first instance whether it is you that has cancer, or someone close you need to get over the initial shock. Cancer patients wake up at three in the morning thinking that maybe it will have all gone away as if by magic. But it won't. It never does.

There is no point in bottling it up. Men in particular tend to keep everything to themselves. I've dealt with male patients who didn't even tell their wives or partners they had cancer. It's never my place to comment on their marriage – and I'd hardly claim to be qualified to myself – but that is hardly healthy. You need someone to talk to and to help you get through this.

Once the news has been broken to you by your physician, you need to identify who it is who is going to work with you in getting through to the other side. If you are married, then your partner is the most obvious person. But not everyone is married or has a partner. If you are divorced, or widowed, perhaps one of your children would be the most obvious person. Of course, they may be very busy. Cancer afflicts the elderly most of all, and the children of the patients are usually grown up themselves, with children and jobs to worry about. Some patients will worry about being a burden. Don't. Your children won't be happy if you die because you didn't want to take up their time making sure you got the best treatment available. If you have no children, and no partner, then a close friend would be best. Again, don't be embarrassed to ask for help. The rule is simple. Don't try and do this by yourself. Beating cancer is not a solo mission.

Most healthcare systems will offer you cancer counsellors to help you in the weeks immediately after your cancer has been diagnosed. I don't want to disparage counsellors. Many of them do an excellent job. Nearly all of them are sympathetic, caring people. But you shouldn't rely on them.

First, and most obviously, they are not medically trained. They are there to help you emotionally, but they won't be able to guide you through the vast range of different treatments available. Of course, emotional support is helpful. But it isn't going to deal with your cancer – only medical care can do that.

Second, and perhaps more importantly, they are part of the system. They are within the cancer industry. To get the best care possible, as we have already seen, you are going to have to manipulate that system. The counsellor isn't going to help you to do that – it's not part of their training, and neither is it in their interests.

In fact, the best way of coping with cancer is to start taking control. That is what will get you on the track to being cured.

Once you've identified the person who is going to help you through this – your partner, your son or daughter or a friend – the next thing you have to do is to equip yourself with the maximum amount of information possible.

That is the key – you have to understand exactly what it is you have and how it is going to be fixed.

To start with, you need to know precisely what kind of cancer it is you are suffering from.

You should ask your physician for a copy of your pathology report, and also any imaging that has been done. You are entitled to that. Don't start shouting at people or snapping at people about your rights. You are going to have to work with the doctors and nurses in your healthcare system over the next few months, and you won't get anywhere by being rude. If they don't like you, they will very quickly find ways of making sure you go to the back of the queue. Just politely ask. They won't offer it to you – but they won't say no either.

Of course, you may not be able to understand it at first. Medicine has its own language – and it is double Dutch to most people. The first thing you do at medical school is learn a whole new vocabulary. Once you get the hang of it, it is, like any language, easy enough. But to outsiders it can be baffling, and often deliberately so. But there is usually a bottom line, and that is what you need to go straight to. It will tell you most of what you need to know.

It is the most useful document you can have. When I see a patient for a second opinion, the first thing I do is ask for the pathology report. It will tell me almost everything I need to know.

People often ask me whether a second opinion is really worthwhile. In my experience, the initial diagnosis is very rarely wrong. In less than 5% of cases will the assessment be radically changed. What will help you, however, is talking to your doctor, and getting a better idea of the range of treatments available to you.

Nor will positive thinking help you very much. You may read articles in the papers about people 'beating cancer' through willpower, or a positive mental attitude. Don't be taken in by it. What really beats cancer is the right medical treatment delivered at the right time. But positive thinking can help in one respect. It will help you to get organised, and to find the treatment that you really need.

What will help you, as I said earlier, is taking control of the situation.

Doctors are not used to being challenged. The more senior the doctor, the more likely that is to be true. Hospitals are every bit as hierarchical as the Army in their own way, and a senior consultant is no more used to having his opinions second-guessed than is a General. At first, he or she may not like it very much. But if you say from the start that you would like to get a second opinion, and that you want to have all the treatment options explained to you in language you can understand, then fairly quickly they will get used to you.

Right from the start, you need to get the treatment plan worked out – that is the most important thing to get right.

There is no shortage of places to go for more information. Most obviously, people start with the internet.

The last time I checked there were more than a billion cancer sites listed on Google. By the time you read this book, there will probably be several million more.

Of course, the web can't always be trusted. No one checks or verifies most of the material that's posted on websites, and you can't always be sure it is accurate. You have to bear in mind as well that someone has put up the website for a reason. They are usually trying to sell something, whether it is medicines, or insurance, or books. You need to be aware of what they are trying to sell.

But that said there are some really excellent and informative websites out there. In the UK, the Cancer Research www.cancerresearchuk.org and the Macmillan Cancer Support www.macmillan.org.uk sites are probably the best two. They will be the best starting point, and both organisations have put a huge effort into making sure they offer you accurate information.

In the US, you should definitely visit www.cancer.gov. It is one of the best sites in the world, and although it is pitched mainly at US based patients, it is also a very useful resource for anyone in the world. Then there is www.cancer.org the excellent and informative site of the American Cancer society. And finally, there is the National Cancer Centre Network site with detailed guidelines for a wide range of cancers at www.nccn.org. Between them these five websites give you the most accurate practical information together with links to lots of other accredited sites. There are many other very good sites in many countries that are very useful. But there are also some dreadful ones that tout all sorts of dramatic cures for cancer. Avoid getting sucked into them without a critical eye.

You should take your pathology report, and then go to one of the main, well-respected websites, and spend a few hours really understanding what kind of cancer you have, and what the options for treatment are.

Don't be afraid of looking at the prognosis. The survival rates for some cancers are quite high, and for others unfortunately very low. At first, it may come as a terrible shock to learn that the chance of your living through the next two years is perhaps as little as 30%. But you should bear in mind that doctors are always too cautious in their assessments. Just because the chances of survival are low, there is no reason why you shouldn't be the one who pulls through.

I've had patients during my career who all the medical experts would have said had zero chance of surviving another year, and yet, twenty years later, are walking around leading perfectly happy lives. What was different about them, and why they survived when others didn't, I don't know. There was no medical explanation that I could see, and neither was there anything very different about their personality. It was just one of those mysteries we can't really explain.

So don't be afraid to look up your chances of survival. And don't be dismayed by what you see.

Remember, if this book has a key message, it is that equipping yourself with the maximum amount of information possible, and taking control of your treatment, are the two keys to beating your cancer. And you can't make a start on either if you are not prepared to face up to news that may be distressing. Just remember the young man in Seat 20B.

Chapter Twelve: What's the receptionist called?

How to be a welcome patient and get the system to work for you

Pause for a moment and think what it is like to be a receptionist in a cancer centre. It's a low-paid job, and you'll be earning about the minimum wage, or only slightly more. You might have had other ambitions, but for one reason or another they haven't worked out, and now you're stuck in a job where you have no real prospects of promotion.

The place is full of well qualified doctors, nurses and technicians, all of whom earn far more money than you do, and sometimes work shorter hours as well, but who treat you with very little respect, and are sometimes downright rude. They don't even know your name.

In short, your daily life can be a struggle.

And then, to cap it all, the hospital computer has crashed yet again today and everybody will just have to wait to get their next appointment sorted. Then some idiot with cancer starts shouting at you in a very unpleasant way because his CT scan hasn't been booked at precisely the time they expected.

So how are you going to respond?

Move his or her case up to the top of the queue? Make sure the imaging centre magically finds some extra time tomorrow and can book in another appointment. Or quietly move that person's file to the back of the system, and silently hope that they die before they come back to harass you again?

The people working in the healthcare system – even in a very bureaucratic system such as Britain's NHS – are nearly all good people. They are kind, well-meaning, and good at empathising with the suffering of others. In many ways, it is a self-selecting system. Heartless, cold-blooded, rapacious and cut-throat characters, who'd sell their own grandmothers for a few pounds, get themselves jobs as bond traders or venture capitalists, not as doctors, nurses or receptionists.

But there is one simple thing it is worth learning as soon as you step into the cancer system.

They are not saints.

And they won't respond well if you are not polite to them.

You need to get the staff you will be dealing with on your side – and that starts with the most humble of them, the person who greets you at the front desk.

As we have discussed in the earlier chapters, the cancer industry is a system. And while it has an interest in curing cancer patients generally – if it didn't it wouldn't stay in business very long – but it doesn't make much difference whether you are one of the people who get cured or not.

That is particularly true in a public sector system such as the NHS, where you are not even a customer. It really makes no difference what your experience is like. Everyone gets paid the same and no one loses their job if things go wrong. But it's also true as well in private systems. Some patients will get excellent care and some very poor care. And it doesn't make much difference to the people running the system whether you are one of the patients who are treated well or badly. But it makes a big difference to you.

The trick is to get the system working in your interests. And one of the constant themes of this book is to show you how to do that.

The first thing to do is to start by inverting the pyramid.

You probably think of the cancer system as run by a consultant, with some of the junior doctors underneath him, and then a whole layer of nurses and other clinical specialists' underneath those and finally the receptionists and support staff right at the bottom of the whole structure. Get on well with the consultant – the person right at the very top of the pyramid – and you probably imagine you'll get the whole system working for you.

But actually, it would be better to do it the other way around. Get the people at the bottom of the pyramid on your side and you will very quickly find that your whole experience is transformed – and your chances of living through this will be dramatically improved.

Start with the receptionist. As I said, she is almost certainly lowly-paid, and may well have thwarted ambitions or a difficult home life as well. But she will be a fundamentally well-meaning person. Treat her kindly, and with respect, and make sure that you are always polite and friendly.

Do the same with the consultant's secretary. Again, she is relatively poorly paid and is under a lot of pressure as all healthcare systems are trying to save money. Outsourcing of dictated reports and letters using telephones to Asia has become commonplace to try and reduce the number of secretaries employed in our NHS. Whilst the work is of good quality – it's typed in Asia but printed in the hospital in the UK – it depersonalizes the whole business of communication. She will often feel swamped with endless bits of paper. But she can be a very powerful ally in your care. She needs to be made to feel good somehow.

Get to know their names, and always use them. And give her a small gift.

You don't want to go overboard. I remember treating an Omani patient once at Hammersmith Hospital. She was a very nice lady, and her treatment had gone reasonably well, but I hadn't done an outstanding or exceptional job – I had just given her the same treatment any doctor would have given to a patient with her condition. At the end, she slipped £500 into the top pocket of my white coat.

That was very nice. I'd certainly be pleased if all my patients did that – and I'd be a lot richer as well. But money is not appropriate, and certainly not in the UK. The doctors and nurses are already being paid for doing their job and they don't expect to receive anything extra from the patients.

What will work perfectly for you is to give the receptionist a bunch of flowers, a bottle of wine, or a box of chocolates. Wait until the third or fourth appointment so you already know her a bit, and at that point make a small gesture to thank her for her help. Don't be too generous. That will just embarrass everyone – a bottle rather than a case of wine is just right.

Choose a gift that seems appropriate – and the more thoughtful the better.

At my hospital, we treated a woman for many years that ran a greengrocery shop. And every few months when she came for follow up visits after her cancer had been treated she would bring in a fabulous box of fresh fruit for all the staff. They loved it – the contents were so much better than supermarket fruit. And the whole team felt good. When our patient developed symptoms suggesting a possible recurrence she was sorted out instantly.

Make a simple gesture such as that, and you'll find it makes a big difference.

In most cancer centres, receptionists and secretaries have a power that most patients don't really understand. They control the flow of appointments. They organise the agenda. They make sure that everything happens at the right time – or, of course, at the wrong time if they don't like you very much.

So, getting to know them, and getting them on your side, is the first rule of being a successful cancer patient. It will automatically move you to the top of the queue.

Next, try and see the same person every time. As a cancer patient, you are likely to need regular blood tests, maybe several scans, and perhaps several courses of chemotherapy. You are going to be seeing a lot of specialist medical staff. Try and make sure you see the same nurse of doctor each time you go. Just ask. If you don't, you'll just be allocated the next person who happens to be on the rota that day, but if you make a point of requesting a particular person, you will usually be allowed to. That way you can build up a rapport with them. As they get to know you, they will care about your treatment more, and make sure everything goes smoothly. It is a small thing – but it can make a big difference.

I remember as though it was yesterday a patient who always got the 09.00 am slot in my Monday clinic. I'm pretty punctual so she was away by 09.15 and saw me personally not a registrar. I found out she got this appointment every time by sending my secretary post cards and at Christmas a bottle of wine. In all honesty she was an interesting and cheerful lady and always a pleasure to see. She was pleasant to the right person that controlled the system.

The second rule is to be patient. I have seen terrible examples of rudeness towards patients, particularly in the NHS. In one cancer centre where I was visiting to give a lunchtime lecture I sat for a few minutes in the radiotherapy waiting area. I remember a single, over-worked and very hassled receptionist, on the phone constantly, probably organising her social life, with a sheaf of papers spread out untidily across her desk, clearly ignoring the eight elderly patients standing uncomfortably in a queue waiting to organise their treatment. Alongside her was a grossly overweight staff nurse stuffing herself on chips in a polystyrene take-away from the hospital canteen watching Wimbledon on TV and ignoring the patients.

It was terrible – the NHS at its soul-destroying, semi-Communist worst. And things like that just shouldn't happen.

And yet, in any kind of healthcare system, whether it is private or state-funded, well or badly-managed, you will have to learn to wait sometimes.

There is a reason why sick people are called patients. Because they have to learn to be patient. Actually, the derivation of patient comes from the same source as pathology – the study of suffering. At Easter the Christian church has paschal candles to represent the suffering of Christ. In a modern world the word patient seems terribly politically incorrect. Gone are cancer sufferers and victims – instead we have people living with cancer. It's only a matter of time before the word patient is consigned to the dustbin.

Every healthcare system has pressures in it. Unless there is massive over-capacity, there will inevitably be some waiting around. Be prepared for it, and it won't be so stressful. For example, if you have a 4.00 pm appointment, don't assume you can make an important business meeting at 5.00 pm. It might not be possible. Cutting things too fine will make you stressed and angry, and that won't help anyone. Allow at least two or three hours out of your day for your appointment. Bring a book, and if you have to wait an hour to see the doctor just accept that's the way things are.

Don't get angry with the staff. It won't make things move any quicker – and it certainly won't make you any more popular.

But at the same time don't be a pushover. The one key message of this book is that the most important person in managing your cancer treatment is you. You need to think about the problems that might come up – and work out in advance how you are going to deal with them.

So, what kind of issues might you face? And how should they be tackled in the right way. The most common one is an unreasonable delay in your treatment.

There are lots of steps you are going to have to go through. Blood tests will have to be done, images made, reports prepared, and even once that is done you may need repeated sessions of chemotherapy or surgery.

It is important that it all happens at the right time. The difference between treating a cancer quickly and delaying for a few months can quite literally be life or death. Of course, no one is going to get everything they need immediately. Unless the system is built with vast spare capacity, that just isn't possible – and as we've already seen, cancer care is already expensive enough as it is. Some waiting is perfectly acceptable. But too much can be fatal. If you sense that is happening, first find out who is the person who is meant to be delivering your service. You don't need to write to the consultant in charge of your treatment in the first instance. Simply find out who the right person is and politely tell them that your treatment might be a little behind schedule.

Right at the start of your treatment you should have worked out a rough timetable of your care, so you should know what to expect at each stage of the process. And if you use the websites at the end of this book, you will have all the information you need to check whether your cancer is being treated in the most effective way.

Don't get into a state about a delay of a few days. It won't make much difference one way or another. But if it stretches into weeks or even months, then make it clear that you are aware the schedule is slipping, and something needs to be done. Usually, a simple letter to the specialist in charge will move everything along very quickly. Only if that doesn't work do you need to take matters up with someone more senior – but ninety percent of the time it will work.

You should think about how your behaviour shapes what the people treating you think of you – and how much they want to help. You don't want to become what doctors often refer to as a 'heart-sink' patient – meaning our hearts sink every time you step into the room.

I remember one patient, who happened to be a journalist on a well-known national newspaper. He had leukaemia, so we all understood that he was in a terrible state, both mentally and physically. Things were not going well for him. He came for an appointment at the hospital and got into a huge argument about a space in the car park, and started shouting at a man who he thought had pinched his place. Now, I agree that the person should have let him have the space. I certainly would have. But the fact is that he didn't. The two men ended up shouting and swearing at each other, and then getting into a fight. My patient arrived for his appointment with blood on his face! We had to get him treatment for that before we could even start worrying about his cancer. He wasn't a big man, and in his condition, a fight was the last thing he needed. To make matters worse, he then wrote a piece in the following week's Sunday paper he worked for about how terrible his cancer treatment had been at the hospital mentioning my name. Needless to say, that didn't make him at all popular with the staff or myself.

Remember just because you have cancer doesn't mean the world is going to start rearranging itself to suit you. There aren't any parking spaces reserved for cancer patients – maybe there should be, but there aren't. You are still going to get speeding tickets; you will still get stuck in traffic jams and your children are still going to cause all the same kind of problems as they always have. None of the other problems in your life are about to magically disappear just because of your illness. You need to learn how to cope with all the challenges that everyday life throws up – as well as having cancer.

Another common problem is that things just don't happen the way they are meant to. Forms start getting lost. Appointments are not made. Tests don't get scheduled.

The truth is the cancer centre is an office like any other office. Not everyone is competent, and not everyone is keeping their eye on the ball – it is just that the stakes are a lot higher for the customer (or patient). The system is not necessarily efficient, and where more of it is controlled by the state, the less efficient it is likely to be.

Do something about it.

It is no good just accepting that mistakes will be made. And don't imagine that your consultant will sort it out. They're busy as well – and not necessarily keeping their eye on the ball either.

Write to the person in charge and ask why things aren't happening according to schedule. Usually, a simple reminder will be enough. The issue will be quickly resolved. But if it isn't, you can always write to the consultant as well.

A third common problem is that you won't be getting the treatment you think you should be getting.

You might be looking at the websites, and you'll see that many patients get treatment

Y for cancer X. And you'll start wondering why you aren't getting that treatment. The first rule is, don't panic.

In truth, there are often two different treatments for the same kind of cancer, and both are equally valid. For breast cancer, for example, you might have surgery and then you might have chemotherapy or radiotherapy or both. Different consultants will reach different conclusions based on factors such as the age of the patient, their other medical conditions and how advanced the cancer is. Your doctor may simply have decided on what they believe is the best treatment for you.

But that doesn't mean you have to accept it. Oncologists are no more infallible than any other class of professional. They make judgements based on the available evidence, but that doesn't mean it is always the right judgement.

Ask questions. If you think you should be getting treatment Y rather than treatment X, ask for an explanation. Don't be rude or threatening, and most of all don't start screaming about your rights. Just discuss it in an informed and intelligent way. There may well be a very good reason why you are not getting that treatment. And once you've heard it, you may well be satisfied.

The most important lesson is to remember that your cancer unit is just another office staffed by on the whole fairly competent human beings but who will have a lot of other things going on in their life apart from treating your cancer. Understand how it functions, figure out what the pressures are, and make sure you present yourself in the way that ensures you get the best treatment possible.

And don't forget to get on well with the receptionist. And the consultant's secretary. At least know their first names.

Chapter Thirteen: Taking the midnight flight

Learn how you can unblock delays by being proactive

We've all been on airline websites. You're planning a trip to Rome for a couple of days. Perhaps it's your wedding anniversary or maybe you are planning a short mini-break with someone you've just met. You scroll down the list of flights. There is a plane leaving at seven o'clock on Friday evening. Just enough time to get out of the office if you sneak away a little early, get up to the airport, and get through security. You should be relaxing on the Piazza Navona with a drink before midnight, with two whole days ahead of you, before catching the seven o'clock flight home on Sunday night, arriving in time to catch some sleep before returning to work on Monday morning.

Perfect.

There's just one catch.

Everyone else thinks those times are perfect it as well. And because of that, the flights are very, very expensive.

And as you scroll down, you'll notice that other flights are much cheaper. The Wednesday morning flight is significantly less, for example. So is the Tuesday afternoon one. And there is a flight at midnight on Monday night which will cost you less then the glass of wine you'll order when you get to the other end.

Of course, it's a lot less convenient. But with the money you save on the flight, you could stay in a five-star hotel rather than a two-star one or stay for four nights rather than two. And, depending on how flexible you can be with your time, and how much you value convenience, you can make a choice one way or the other.

Of course, having cancer is not much like a weekend in Rome – it's not nearly so much fun for starters. But actually, the economics of the two industries are not so very different.

Think about that airline. It has to buy a bunch of planes, and there isn't much change out of $80 million even for a fairly small aircraft such as an Airbus 320. That is an expensive piece of kit. It has to employ pilots, and cabin crew, and book slots at airports, deal with security, create a website and have ticketing systems. A lot of money has to be spent. And once that money is spent, it has to work the equipment as hard as possible to make a return on its investment. So, it is worth offering those midnight flights on Monday at a bargain price even if it only just covers the cost of the fuel – because most of its costs are fixed, and it might as well make a little bit of money, whilst making big profits on those Friday evening flights.

The cancer industry is much the same. There is a lot of very expensive kit involved. An MRI scanner for example won't leave you any change out of £1 million and could cost a lot more. True, it is not as much as a new Boeing or Airbus, but it's still a lot of money. And you need to keep it working as hard as possible to make it worth spending that much money on a single piece of machinery.

People usually all want their scans at the same time. Three o'clock on a Wednesday afternoon. Ten o'clock on a Monday morning. Those are the popular time slots.

But if you are willing to go off-peak, you can get it done a lot cheaper.

Whatever kind of healthcare system you are in, whether it's private or public, is going to have some kind of rationing involved – although for all the reasons we have discussed, no one will ever publicly admit it. They won't always give you all the scans you need simply because there isn't the capacity in the system and it would cost an absolute fortune if they offered them to everyone.

So why not just pay for it yourself? Is this a heresy?

People are put off paying for things themselves because they think it is going to cost them a fortune. But while medicine is undoubtedly expensive, some top-ups to your cancer treatment are not actually going to bankrupt someone who has been working for most of their lives and has some reasonable level of savings.

And if you haggle, it will cost you much less.

Say you want an additional scan for example to see whether your chemotherapy is making progress in treating your cancer, but your health provider is not willing to provide it until the course of treatment is complete. Get a friend or a family member to phone around. You will find there is somewhere within most major cities that can offer you that service privately. Call them up and ask them how much it costs, and when they tell you, ask them if they can do it for a bit less if you come at an off-peak time. It is no different from haggling over the price of a hotel room – or that airline ticket.

An MRI scan might cost you £500–£700 – a significant sum of money, but not that much to set against the cost of curing your cancer. And that price will come down if you get it done at the weekend.

There are other things you might want to pay for.

A blood test for example should only cost you about £20. There isn't much point in haggling over that because it is a relatively minor sum. But if you feel you need it to check the rate of progress in dealing with your cancer, and if it is not being offered as frequently as you like by your doctors, there is no reason not to pay for one yourself.

A second opinion might also be worth paying for. There is no automatic right to a second opinion within the NHS, although people often think that there is. But it is often a good way of setting your mind at ease and making sure that you know you are getting the right treatment. In the UK, that will cost around £300. There is no point in haggling over it because it is a fairly standard fee that any specialist will charge for a private consultation. Again, it is not the kind of sum that is going to break the bank for most people. If you feel you need it, there is no reason not to pay for it yourself.

In my experience, 90% of second opinions agree completely with the first opinion. In five percent of the cases, there might be a minor change in treatment recommended.

In a final five percent of cases, there might be a radical change of treatment prescribed.

Of course, if you are one of those five percent you are going to have a difficult decision to make. One consultant is going to be recommending one way of treating your cancer. And another one is going to be recommending a completely different course of action.

Both of them will no doubt be perfectly well qualified in their fields, with lots of credentials, and many years of experience of treating cancer patients.

You probably won't have the experience to make an informed decision.

The point to bear in mind is, as I said at the start of this chapter, everything is negotiable. Doctors are not unapproachable, and they rarely have closed minds. They know that cancer treatment is as much an art as a precise science. Explain to both doctors that you have received conflicting opinions and talk through with them why they have reached that precise judgement about the best way to deal with your cancer. After that, talk it through with them, preferably in the company of a friend or a family member. It is often quite legitimate for different courses of treatment to be prescribed. In the end, it will be up to you to decide. But you should do so based on having all the information available.

One of the things that will be hardest to negotiate is the cost of drugs – although it may well be one of the most expensive parts of the treatment of your cancer and the one that is most likely to be rationed by your healthcare provider.

As we saw earlier, over the last decade there have been dozens of new cancer drugs released onto the market. Many of them are very useful. Over the next decade there will probably be many more. There have been huge advances in out understanding of how to treat the disease with pharmaceuticals, and the fruits of all that research in the laboratories are only now coming through. But they are all very expensive. And one of the ways that governments and insurers try and keep the cost of cancer care under control is by restricting the availability of the most expensive drugs.

You shouldn't believe everything you read in the papers or on the internet. The drug companies and their cheerleaders are always hyping up the effectiveness of some new medicine on the market. That is how they make their money. It may well be that the experts in your healthcare system have decided that a particular drug is not worth the cost, or the side-effects, and so have decided not to prescribe it for perfectly legitimate reasons. You should not assume that you are not getting a new wonder drug you have read about simply because your healthcare provider wants to save money.

Sometimes, however, that will be the case. You will be denied a drug that would help treat your cancer because it is too expensive.

Of course, in those circumstances you may to some very small degree be sympathetic. Maybe it's the case that not everyone can be prescribed this very expensive drug without bankrupting the whole system. But it is unlikely you will be selfless enough to accept that argument on anything other than a theoretical level. If you need the drug, you want it to be prescribed for you, As I said right at the start, you only get one life. Maybe the costs of cancer care do need to be contained, but not at your expense.

So, what should you do?

In the first instance do talk to your consultant. As in so many other examples we have discussed, simply being an informed, well-organised, and polite but a determined patient, can make a huge difference to your care. Most healthcare systems are not absolute. There are usually back doors and exceptions, and if you make it clear you are aware of the drug you need, and why you need it, you might find that it becomes available. As in so many other areas of life, if you don't' ask you don't get – cancer drugs are no exception to that rule.

In the UK, as we have seen, there is the Cancer Drug Fund. It is a big pit of money the government has set up to fund the supply of specialist cancer drugs. Not many people know about it. If you ask for the drugs you believe you need to be supplied by the Fund, you may well successful.

Many other countries have similar schemes, either paid for by the government, or by charitable foundations. Find out what they are, and whether you qualify.

You can also go to court.

On several occasions, I have appeared as an expert witness where a patient has taken a decision to deny them access to a cancer drug to judicial review. I sat in the public gallery during much of the hearing of one such case. It was fascinating to listen to the arguments on both sides. Watching lawyers argue on clinical decisions in their wigs and gowns in a stuffy Victorian courthouse was a surreal experience. The cost of the hearing would have provided at least 6 patients the optimal treatment.

But I am not really sure it is worthwhile. In that instance – which the lady I appeared for won – the cost of arguing the case in court would have paid for ten people to have been prescribed the drug. And that would have certainly been a better use of public money.

And the woman in question became obsessed with getting the treatment to the detriment of her psychological health.

Unfortunately, she had a severe cancer, and she was not going to live much longer whether she had the drug or not. True, the medicine was going to prolong her life a little. But she spent much of her last year of life fighting a bitter battle through the courts rather than spending more time with her family or travelling or doing any of the things that would have made the time left to her more pleasurable and fulfilling.

In the end, I was not really sure it was a worthwhile for her to take the case so far. But in the end that is a judgement that every patient will have to make.

Finally, should you consider paying for the drug yourself?

This is always a difficult decision, and one that any specialist in cancer is going to be asked at some point in their career – and probably with increasing frequency as the number of very costly drugs on the market increases.

There is no right or wrong answer.

It depends to some degree on the financial position of the patient. If you are a multi-millionaire, of course you are going to pay for it. That's a no-brainer. Likewise, a very poor person simply isn't going to be able to pay for the medicine. So that doesn't require much thought either. But most people are somewhere in the middle, where the choices are rather harder. Cancer drugs are expensive, but not off-the-planet expensive. A six-month course of a drug might cost you as much as a new car for example. It is a big financial decision and not one to be taken lightly. But most people have a car. They can raise the money if they really need it – and as I said earlier, you only get one life.

It also depends on the drug, and on how advanced the cancer is. If it's only going to prolong your life by a few weeks and even then in great physical discomfort, then perhaps it is not worth it. You might be better off spending time with your family or making sure your husband or wife, your partner or your children are well cared for after you're gone.

But if the drug, perhaps in combination with chemotherapy or surgery, stands a good chance of permanently eradicating your cancer, then it is definitely something you'd want to consider. Between those two extremes many drugs might well prolong your life by several years and allow you to have a reasonably high quality of life as well. In which case, it might well be worth considering paying for the drug yourself – assuming of course that you can't get your healthcare provider to pay for it. If it means cutting back on other expenditures, then so be it.

These are hard decisions. One thing you should do is make sure you are getting the best possible deal. Drug prices will usually be the same across the country, but prescription policies in the UK for example may vary by country because different health authorities may have different policies in the prescription of particular drugs. There is nothing to stop you registering as a patient in a different part of the country if that means you may get the medicine you need. Drugs prices can vary dramatically between different countries. Use the internet to find out if you can get the same medicine sent to you from somewhere else at a much lower cost. Canada, for example, often has much lower prices.

You may find you can get precisely the same drug at 30% less than you could get it at home – and if so, that is going to make paying for your own prescription a lot more affordable. You have to be careful, naturally. And it is something you should only do in close consultation with your physician. Many of the websites you find on Google will not be selling proper drugs at all, but cheap copies, or else phoney medicines that are downright dangerous. But just because there are some scammers out there does not mean that there are not some legitimate sites as well. You probably feel comfortable buying books, wine or airline tickets on the internet without worrying that you are being scammed or ripped off and there is no real reason by you shouldn't be buying medicines as well.

That is the theme of this chapter – and in many ways of this whole book.

Everything is negotiable. And it is up to you to take control of your own cancer treatment – not leave it entirely up to the professionals.

Chapter Fourteen: Life after cancer

Learning to live with uncertainty and yet get back to normal

It may be hard to imagine that life goes on after cancer. Many people undergo treatment while they are still experiencing the initial shock of diagnosis. When this is over, their attempt to return to normal life is often an uphill struggle. For most people and their families, the experience of cancer, whatever its outcome, will change their lives forever. Their values may be realigned and their whole perspective on life will be changed. The intensity of pleasure, sadness and emotions, becomes much greater. It is important in this process that patients and families do not become victims.

Although at first it is hard to view anything with a long-term perspective, restoration to a full emotional life is every bit as important as successful therapy. If the price of cure is isolation and fear, nobody will benefit. Many believe that when their treatment course has been finished – and it may have been an arduous one in terms of number of visits and side effects – they will go to a follow-up clinic where they will be told that they are cured. This approach is upheld by the media that often talk about celebrities and their relatives "beating cancer" very rapidly after treatment has been completed.

Unfortunately, cancer is not like that. By the time it has been discovered there are usually more than a billion cancer cells in the body. The vast majority of these cells will have disappeared during treatment but present-day screening techniques mean that we cannot detect even as many as 10,000 cells accurately. As a result, any doctor who tells a patient as little as one month after treatment they have been cured, is being inappropriately optimistic. It may be very likely that they have been cured but a definite statement is not possible at this stage.

Follow-up clinics are very useful both for you and your doctors. It sometimes takes a bit of time to cease dreading these occasions but as gaps between clinic visits increase, so reassurance comes. The clinic is there as a safety-net to which you can return if your symptoms recur of if your fears about the disease become overwhelming. You will be asked about new symptoms, examined usually just in the area of the body that is relevant to the type of cancer you've been treated for and then some blood tests, x-rays or other tests may be carried out.

As we learn more about cancer, it is becoming apparent that fewer of the tests rather than more are indicated. In the vast majority of cancers, we do not have reliable ways of following up patients and discussing whether they have relapsed or developed microscopic disease away from the site of the original tumour. In those cancers where any recurrence or spread of the disease is likely to respond well to treatment and where there are sensitive tests that can detect recurrent disease, these will be done to ensure that any problems are detected at an early stage. For these types of cancer, blood tests, x-rays and scans are important and will be a regular part of the patient's review.

In many situations tests will not be carried out unless there are obvious worrying symptoms. You should not feel necessarily neglected simply because investigations are not performed. Discuss the situation and also whether it is worth pursuing at your own expense a special test to ensure that things are going well. Follow-up is usually carried out for at least five years and sometimes for life in certain cancers. The five year cut-off is based on patterns of survival in people that have been successfully treated for cancer. We know that at five years, if a patient is alive with most types of cancer and has not shown any signs of recurrence, it is likely that they have been cured. This can be calculated from life tables used by actuaries in the insurance industry. You compare a group of people that have had cancer with an age-matched controlled group that have not, then when the survival curves become parallel, cure has effectively been obtained. Of course, this only looks at large sets of patients, not you as an individual.

Getting back to work

The diagnosis of cancer is likely to be followed by your life being taken over by a series of visits for tests, surgery, radiotherapy and possibly six months of chemotherapy. The point at which you are well enough to return to work varies enormously depending on the type of treatment and the way it is affecting you. It also depends to a certain extent on your job. Your GP or family doctor can advise about any benefits or financial support to which you may be entitled. Once employers are aware of the reasons for your absence, they may have their own ideas about your subsequent ability to do your job.

It is essential to enlist the support and help of your medical staff at this point. Any specific disability can be anticipated. If certain tasks associated with the job are impossible, it may be feasible to amend your job so that you can cope. However there is no reason why the majority of people with cancer cannot resume full-time employment exactly as before if they've had a chance to regain their strength. Getting back to work is the most important factor in returning to normal life and much of your self-esteem is likely to depend on this. If you have any specific difficulties in relation to your job or employer, you should air these in the clinic. An explanatory letter from the doctor will often do much to dispel any fears and misconceptions. It is not only patients with cancer who fear the disease; its taboos extend to people close to the person. Irrational behaviour from family, friends and work colleagues is not unusual and the only way this can be countered is to avoid mystery and replace it with transparency and understanding.

Recurrent disease

The ultimate fear of most patients is that their cancer will come back. As time goes by, so the risk of recurrence decreases and your follow-up visits to the clinic will become less frequent. Of course, the chances of recurrence depend on what type of cancer you have and how it had spread when you were first treated. Some highly aggressive cancers will probably recur within two years of diagnosis if they are going to recur at all. And if you've been disease-free for five years, it is likely that you have been cured.

On the other hand, there are diseases that respond to primary treatment and many years later, sometimes decades, cells that have spread from the primary site begin to grow, causing problems again. Many cancers, probably up to half, can still be cured at the time of the diagnosis of recurrence. These include those sensitive to hormone therapy, such as breast and prostatic cancer, and those that can be cured by chemotherapy, lymphomas and testicular tumours or those where the only problems are local recurrence, which can be dealt with by further surgery or radiotherapy.

Although some cancers cannot be cured, this may not in fact reduce the patient's life expectancy. Many patients live with their cancer for many years. If they are in their mid-sixties when they get cancer, it is possible to reach the sprightly age of eighty and still be in good shape even though the disease has slowly recurred. It is also important to maintain a balance between the length of time you can survive and the quality of life. Getting obsessed about the cancer so it drives all social activity out of your life is not a good idea. If the disease does come back then there will be options ranging from no further treatment, through to trying banded chemotherapy regimens or in some cases experimental treatment for clinical treatment. Remember that the final decision is yours and yours alone.

If you are offered a new drug on a clinical trial determine the likely benefits before rushing into taking something just because it is there or because your doctor has persuaded you that it is in your best interests. Identify exactly the nature of the treatment being offered and read widely about it on the internet. Go back and ask the trial co-ordinator for more details about the various treatment arms. It may be a randomized trial out of which you will get nothing of any benefit. Ultimately all of us have to die, although we fear it enormously. Gradually as we make cancer a chronic controllable illness, we'll be pushing it further out as a cause of death into old age and so the whole process will be less frightening. But you are in charge of when you want to stop treatment; do not be afraid to make that decision.

Chapter Fifteen: The future of cancer care

Peering into the crystal ball

Eventually cancer will become like diabetes, a chronic controllable illness. We may still not be able to cure metastatic cancer, but we will keep it under control for long periods of time, even thirty years. So, if we look at the delivery of cancer therapy in the future, how will it be done? Well, it will be closer to patients' homes. We won't need hospitals, just a comfortable hotel. Cancer hotels will be the places that will deliver the chemotherapy of the future. Whether we need radiotherapy and surgery will depend on how good future chemotherapy is and we can't predict that yet. There's simply no way of knowing.

In ten years time, we will be in a much better position to judge. I remember twenty years ago speaking to a medical oncologist who told me "Within twenty years, all your radiotherapy machines will be melted down and the radiographers transformed into chemotherapy nurses." Well, that prediction hasn't come about. Now if we're being honest, we can't really predict what's going to happen from now on. We'll definitely have better information technology to monitor treatment and response.

There will be increasing prevalence of cancer that will give rise to far more co-morbidity. And there'll be more people worried because they're living with uncertainty. This will increase the need for good psychosocial care.

We already have a cancer demand pyramid. In every society, rich and poor, there's a core of services that are provided by the equivalent of the NHS at the bottom of the pyramid. There's a line that is wavy because of post-code prescribing above which there is demand but no payment. It's difficult to escape geographical variation with any localised decision-making input on resource rationing. Above the line, there are many unmet demands – complementary medicine, conformal radiotherapy, new drugs, new devices often heavily marketed to the end-consumer through subtle techniques. The line is pushed down by NHS decision-makers – the regulators, NICE, hospital drug committees, Clinical Commissioning Groups, Integrated Care Systems and politicians. They all seek to control spending.

The line is pushed upwards by you the patients, patient advocates, charities and direct to consumer advertising. The industry does a lot covertly for cancer. It's not permitted, so it's hidden. There are no advertisements allowed, but third-party agencies are paid to get stories published in the media implying fantastic benefits from a new drug. They pay grants to patient advocacy movements to push the line up on their behalf. Breast, lung, and prostate advocacy groups have all benefited from this barbed generosity. The media of course loves the line. Sunday papers are filled with stories about people not getting a cancer drug. And of course, politicians love to stimulate controversy and score points against the opposition in a highly politicised healthcare system.

As we go into the future we simply don't know when we're going to get technological success. Let's look at 10 years on – the year 2033. There are four scenarios based on how successful we are and how much society and individuals are going to be willing to pay. The first is technological success and society somehow finding the costs to meet it, in which case cancer becomes a chronic controllable illness. That's obviously the preferred scenario for 2033. There's another scenario in which we achieve success, but society is not willing to pay the cost. Then we get inequity and of course it will vary in different societies around the world. We can see this with HIV in Africa now. If there is little technological success, and if society is willing to pay, we will invest in supportive care. The worst-case scenario is society not willing to pay and no technological success. We then have inequity in the distribution of supportive care and an area where cancer charities can lobby for the less fortunate to make sure that they get good supportive care at the very least.

No scenario leads to immortality of course. We don't like talking about death because we feel uncomfortable. No oncologist likes talking about death, in my experience, because it's a sort of failure and most of us are even frightened to talk about our own mortality. Spending more money on supportive care in its broadest sense will be a good investment with all four futures. What do I think the future is? It's probably somewhere in the middle. It's not going to work out well for every cancer, that's unlikely. The real future is somewhere in the middle, with bits from each scenario. The difficulty now for society is how to deal with this very uncertain future for chemotherapy. The crunch is going to come in the next five years when many of the drugs currently full of hope are scheduled for release onto the market and currently carry huge financial expectations of blockbuster success.

Very little improvement in survival has been achieved by the variations of the local control by permutations of radiation and surgery. Screening may have improved outcomes by shifting patients into earlier stages. We have also improved things by taking the assumption that many apparently localised cancers are advanced and treating them all with additional adjuvant systemic therapy after apparent complete removal by surgery. Intellectually this is, of course, a shambles because we know that the gain from tamoxifen in breast cancer is seen in around 15% of patients, so we're treating 85% of women with tamoxifen for nothing. So, the first advance that is going to come out of our new molecular diagnostics is to use them to select which of localised cancers to leave well alone, after the loco-regional therapy such as surgery or radiotherapy. Personalised treatment pathway planning is the key to the future.

Obviously one of the best ways to shorten the process of evaluating which characteristics in terms of gene and protein patterns are relevant to predict long term success or failure, is to get into archives where we know whether the patient has responded and is dead or alive 20 years later. The whole business of legislation on the protection of human rights and privacy could result in an uphill struggle for this kind of research. Dead people can't give consent to their material being studied. We may have to concentrate much more on the use of surrogate endpoints and biomarkers, detected by imaging or repeat tumour biopsies. We've got to concertina our trials down so that we find more quickly how best to use this extraordinary technology.

Pathology service companies are emerging who have recognised the need for properly consented tissue. Soon all cancer patients will be asked for such consent – it could actually benefit them as well as others. 97% of patients consent for their tissue to be stored when given a full explanation. So, the vast majority of the population actually wish to participate in this activity. We can use Kantian philosophy to argue that if we're a democratic society, it's actually undemocratic for an individual not to release their tissue for the common good of mankind so long as that tissue is of no benefit to them. And pathology laboratories in this country are incinerating vast amounts of tissue every week that could be used for cancer research.

We have defined a certain agenda for chemotherapy but surely there are other areas that are going to be very important between now and 2033? We're going to have more patients who have been treated with more powerful but selective agents and surely, we need to get much more systematic monitoring using new information technology – smart cards and electronic medical records. The renal dialysis service has really set an example of how to do this systematically with every patient. They're measuring patients' urea levels, quality of life and so on. They've shown they can do it and we ought to be doing that in chemotherapy with all cancer drugs, new and old.

Cancer care in 2033 will be driven by the least invasive therapy consistent with long-term survival. Eradication, although still desirable, will no longer be the primary aim of treatment. Cancers will be identified earlier, and the disease process regulated in a similar way to chronic diseases such as diabetes. Surgery and radiotherapy will still have a role but this role may be down-played. How much will depend on the type of cancer a patient has and the stage at which disease is identified. It will also depend on how well the drugs being developed today perform in the future and whether they are best used alone or in combination with these other interventions.

On the other hand, increasing awareness and improved diagnosis will mean there will be a shift towards localised disease, and arguably an increased role for more use of surgery and radiotherapy. In 2023 it is agreed that of one hundred typical cancer patients, around 20 can be cured by simple local surgery. Around 40 have localised disease that can be cured by a combination of surgery and radiotherapy. The remaining 40 patients have disease that has spread, 5 of whom can be considered curable by complex therapies including drugs.

As we move towards 2033, new technologies will enable more of the patients with advanced disease to be treated and controlled but at a price. Surgeons will also find themselves delivering chemotherapy at the time of surgery and will be faced increasingly with the prospect of preventive surgery as people learn more about their predisposition to cancer. In addition, rationing of treatment to the elderly will be less prevalent as drug therapy and surgery become less aggressive and ageism less acceptable to society.

By 2033, cancer treatment will be shaped by a new generation of drugs. What this new generation will look like is not apparent today and will depend on the relative success of agents currently in development. Over the next three to five years, we will understand more fully what benefits these compounds such as the kinase inhibitors are likely to provide. So, what will these drug candidates look like? Today small molecules and monoclonal antibodies are the main focus of research — most of which were designed to target specific gene products that control the biological processes associated with cancer such as signal transduction, angiogenesis, cell cycle control, apoptosis, inflammation, invasion and differentiation. Treatment strategies involving cancer vaccines and gene therapy are also being explored. Although we do not know exactly what these targeted chemotherapeutic agents will look like there is growing confidence that they will work. More uncertain is their overall efficacy at prolonging survival. Many could just provide very expensive palliation. In the future, advances will be driven more by biological understanding of the disease process.

Already we are seeing the emergence of drugs targeted at a molecular level – Herceptin, directed at the HER2 protein, Glivec, which targets the Bcr-Abl tyrosine kinase, and Iressa and Tarceva, directed at EGFR tyrosine kinase. These therapies, and others like them, will be used across a range of cancers. What will be important in 2033 is whether a person's cancer has particular biological or genetic characteristics. Traditional cancer categories will continue to be broken down and genetic profiling will enable treatment to be targeted at the right patients. Patients will understand that treatment options are dependent on their genetic profile. The risks and benefits of treatment will be much more predictable than today.

Clinicians will have access to information that will help them recognise which localised cancers can be left alone, and which tumours will respond to drugs. This will mean fewer patients being exposed to agents with unacceptable toxicity. Such predictive assays will dramatically improve the quality of life for cancer patients. Predictions will never be totally accurate, and patients and doctors will still be faced with uncertainties. However, decisions will be better informed.

Therapies will emerge through our knowledge of the human genome and the use of sophisticated bioinformatics. Targeted imaging agents will be used to deliver therapy at screening or diagnosis. Monitoring cancer patients will also change as technology allows the disease process to be tracked much more closely. Treatment strategies will reflect this and drug resistance will become much more predictable. Biomarkers will allow those treating people with cancer to measure if a drug is working on its target. If it is not, an alternative treatment strategy will be sought. Tumour shrinkage will become less important as clinicians look for molecular patterns of disease.

By 2033, there will be more of a focus on therapies designed to prevent cancer. A tangible risk indicator and risk reducing therapy, along the lines of cholesterol and statins, would allow people to monitor their risk and intervene. Delivering treatment early in the disease process will also be possible because subtle changes in cellular activity will be detectable. This will lead to less aggressive treatment. The role of pharmaceutical companies in the development of new therapies will continue to change. Smaller more specialised companies, such as those in the biotech sector, along with academia, will increasingly deliver drug candidates to the big pharmaceutical companies to market.

In 2033, people will be used to living with risk and will have much more knowledge about their propensity for disease. Already there are posters on London Underground advertising a range of blood tests you can buy without going to your doctor. I predict that consumer diagnostics are the next big thing in medicine. The information technology infrastructure will be available for members of the public to determine their own predisposition to cancer. This in turn will encourage health-changing behaviour and will lead people to seek out information about the treatment options available to them. Patients will also be more involved in decision making as medicine becomes more personalised. Indeed, doctors may find themselves directed by well-informed patients. This, and an environment in which patients are able to demonstrate choice, will help drive innovation towards those who will benefit. However, inequity based on education, wealth and access will continue. You will always have to be pushy to ensure the best care possible.

Clinicians will continue to be concerned about the uncertainty of cancer drugs. Their key questions will be:

- Will the new generation of small molecule kinase inhibitors really make a difference or just be very expensive palliatives?
- How will the drug industry cope with most current high value cytotoxic drugs becoming generic shortly?
- Can expensive late-stage attrition and huge financial waste really be avoided in cancer drug development?
- How will sophisticated molecular diagnostic services be provided?
- Will effective surrogates for cancer preventive agents emerge?
- Will healthy volunteers be used in first-to-man studies?
- Will patient choice involve cost considerations in guiding therapy?

Innovation in cancer treatment

Innovation in cancer treatment is inevitable. However, there are certain prerequisites for the introduction of new therapies. First, innovation has to be translated into usable therapies. These therapies must be deliverable, to the right biological target, and to the right patient in a way that is acceptable by patient, healthcare professional and society. Innovation must also be marketed successfully so that professionals, patients, and those picking up the cost understand the potential benefits. Those making the investment in research will inevitably create a market for innovation even if the benefits achieved are small. The explosion of new therapies in cancer care is going to continue and pricing of these drugs will remain high.

But parallel to this explosion in therapies and increase in costs, a number of confounding factors will make markets smaller. The technology will be there to reveal which patients will not respond to therapy, so making blockbuster drugs history. Doctors will know the precise stage of the disease process at which treatment is necessary. And as cancer transforms into a chronic disease, people will have more co-morbidities, which will bring associated drug-drug interactions and an increase in care requirements.

How do we balance this equation? The pharmaceutical companies will not necessarily want to do the studies to fragment their market. Research leading to rational rationing will need to be driven by the payers of health care. There is a risk that pharmaceutical companies will stop developing drugs for cancer and focus instead on therapeutic areas where there is less individual variation and therefore more scope for profit. Furthermore, development costs are rising. Ten years ago, the average cost of developing a new cancer drug and to get it to market was around $400m. Now it is over $1 billion. At this rate of growth, the cost of developing a new drug in 2033 could be over $2.5bn, an amount unsustainable in a shrinking market. With this in mind, the process of developing drugs will have to be made simpler and faster or nobody will do it.

However, instead of research being made simpler, changes in legislation concerned with privacy and prior consent are making it more difficult. The EU Clinical Trials Directive makes quick hypothesis testing trials impossible. Other challenges exist, as well, such as obtaining consent for new uses of existing human tissue – following political anxiety when consent for removing and storing tissues had not been obtained in the early years of the 21st century. However, surveys have shown that patients who gave consent for tissue to be used for one purpose were happy for it to be used for another. They do not wish to be reminded of their cancer years later. To overcome these constraints regulators will have to start accepting surrogate markers rather than clinical outcomes when approving therapies. Outcome studies may well move to post-registration surveillance of a drug's efficacy similar to cholesterol lowering agents today.

Other factors that will impact on the introduction of new therapies include dampeners such as the National Institute for Clinical Excellence or its equivalent in the early part of the 2020's. Assessing new technologies takes time, even for those with good evidence to support them. There will also be a battle for resources as cancer is transformed into a chronic disease. More people will be receiving preventive drugs as well as long-term therapies. Even if these turn out to be cheap, the numbers of patients involved and the monitoring diagnostics will mean overall costs will rise.

The rise of personalised medicine will mean the temptation to over-treat will disappear. Doctors and patients will know whether a particular treatment is justified. The evidence will be there to support their decisions. As a consequence of this, treatment failure — with all its associated costs — will be less common.

Barriers to introducing new therapies

- The drug industry will continue to compete for investment in a competitive, capitalist environment.
- Fully ethically consented tissue banks will be essential to retrospectively collate value of personalising therapy.
- Blockbuster drugs drive profit – niche products are unattractive in today's market.
- Personalised therapies are difficult for today's industry machine.
- Surrogate endpoints will be essential to register new drugs.
- Novel providers will emerge providing both diagnostic and therapy services.
- Payers will rigidly seek justification for the use of high-cost agents.

Right at the start of this book I said it was likely to be the worst news you would ever have. And, unfortunately, as the years go on, it's news that more and more people are likely to be receiving.

On each working day of this year, over 1,000 people in Britain will be told for the first time that they have cancer. One in three of us will get the disease and the incidence is rising dramatically as our population ages. Cancer predominantly affects the over-60s, although it can strike at any age. There are more over-65s in the world today than have ever reached that age in the past. An ageing population means that the numbers of new cases of cancer diagnosed every year will inevitably rise dramatically. It's the same all over the Western world.

The success of modern medicine at treating infection, heart disease and other illnesses has led to more people living well beyond retirement — and that is certainly a cause for celebration. But this longevity brings new epidemics: cancer, dementia, arthritis, diabetes, frailty, multiple co-morbidities and the inability to cope with independent living.

What we need to is restructure our health and social care systems if we are to deal with this rapid transition.

At the moment, the cost and complexity of cancer care is likely to overwhelm the system. And as it gets more and more expensive, and if, as they may, healthcare systems start to buckle under the strain, then patients are going to have to get a lot smarter at making sure the system works for them.

The first hint that British cancer survival rates were slipping came in 1989, when a series of European comparators, which measured access to cancer treatment and its efficacy, put Britain in last place. I remember a very cross civil servant calling me when my colleagues and I at Hammersmith Hospital pointed this out in our launch for the Cancer Centre Appeal. Kenneth Clarke, the then health minister was seething, as I had spoiled his weekend.

A series of reports by EUROCARE, the pan-European health group, were published three months later which compared cancer survival rates in different nations. The reports concluded that Britain had the worst rates of the wealthier EU countries. A good measure of progress is the number of patients alive five years after initial diagnosis. Different cancers have different five-year survival rates, depending on the effectiveness of treatment. The range is wide: from 98% in testicular cancer to 3% in pancreatic cancer. Britain's results were consistently below the EU average for the four main common cancers: lung, breast, prostate, and colon. Since then, EUROCARE has reported similar findings over the last 20 years. Britain is still the poor man of Europe, while treatments and results in other countries continue to improve. Sure, we are getting better, but we never seem to catch up. If Britain could achieve even the western European average survival rate, it would save the equivalent number of lives as preventing a fully laden jumbo jet crashing at Heathrow every other day. We are still far from being world class.

Cancer care became increasingly politicised in the early 1990s; the initial response of the Conservative government was to form committees. Of these only the Calman-Hine Committee, chaired by the chief medical officer, proved effective, by creating the cancer network that still exists. The others just met for coffee and biscuits.

When Labour came to power in 1997 it was determined to bolster the NHS's cancer capacity. The *NHS Cancer Plan*, launched in 2000, was driven by a huge cash injection into the public sector — the NHS budget tripled, and for cancer care it increased fivefold. Mike Richards, a distinguished oncologist was appointed as the "cancer tsar," and, though his work was admirable, the bureaucracy and politics of the NHS acted to constrain him. Undoubtedly there were improvements, but these have been over-run by increased demand for care, and technological advances in treatments. Cancer patients are becoming more sophisticated in their choices, and the drive is now towards providing a personalised style of medicine. They are pushing for better care and are travelling to get it. One key issue is how to maintain equity in choice and access, both geographically and between different socio-economic groups.

It is essential that all patients should have access to the best new treatments. Powerful new technologies can turn cancer into a chronic disease, which can then be controlled, as with diabetes. A consequence of this is that more people with cancer are living longer, thereby increasing the prevalence of the disease in the population. Rising numbers, increased consumerism and innovation come with a hefty price tag. The current climate of national austerity only makes this problem worse.

Advances in the imaging technology used during surgery to remove primary tumours have minimised the damage done to surrounding tissue, and the increasing use of robotics and keyhole devices means that lengthy stays in hospital are no longer necessary. Radiotherapy has been revolutionised by a combination of sophisticated imaging and computing systems that can contour a tumour accurately. Intensity modulated radiotherapy (IMRT) and image guidance (IGRT) are becoming standard. But in Britain less than 25% of eligible patients have access to these technologies, compared to nearly 100 per cent in France, Germany and Italy.

As we've seen throughout this book the problem with cancer is that it can spread through metastasis. But the molecular revolution has brought a pipeline of new drugs that target receptors and also the molecular cogs that malfunction and which lead to the abnormal growth patterns of a cancer cell. Herceptin was the first drug of this type and has been used to treat breast cancer for the last decade – there are now 1,000 targeted drugs at the trial stage. But, over the last year, the average monthly cost of each of the eight cancer drugs approved in the United States was over $10,000 (£6,000). If this trend continues it could bankrupt the healthcare systems of rich countries and never be affordable by the poor.

Some drugs selectively block tumour blood vessel growth, thereby strangling cancer cells by depriving them of nutrients. Once a cancer has been treated, a new generation of computer tomography and magnetic resonance imaging scanners allow us to monitor progress. Techniques such as positron emission tomography can even provide information on the biochemical changes inside a patient's cancer cells and the new era of cheap DNA and protein analysis of both cancer and normal cells in an individual provides clues as to the best way to treat a cancer.

Computer algorithms, constructed from data from thousands of patients can indicate the best way to reduce disease recurrence. These can suggest appropriate times to administer drugs, hormones and vaccines even when there is no evidence of spread on imaging. The old military metaphors such as the war on cancer, tumour sterilisation and avoiding collateral damage in victims are being replaced by the more peaceful language of disease stabilisation, symbiosis and chronic control with gentle therapies in people living with cancer.

These many improvements have undoubtedly saved lives. But can Britain keep pace with this new world? To do so, we need to look more closely at the fundamental structure of our services to make them more convenient for our customers in the context of their daily lives. The costs of the diagnostics for personalised medicine may be high but the potential for savings enormous. No payer of healthcare is going to ignore this. The days of marketing cancer drugs like a supermarket commodity are over. Developing ways to optimise responses through companion diagnostics and short-term surrogate biomarkers are now going to be essential.

Ultimately there are only three ways to pay for healthcare—tax, insurance, or cash. Being honest with patients about what is available and ensuring equal access is crucial. Honesty about the limits of the NHS's capabilities remains politically sensitive. The use of private funding to provide extra capital has been used for diagnostic equipment and more recently for radiotherapy. But direct involvement of the private sector in whole cancer pathways of care has so far not occurred despite some ambitious attempts.

Until now, patients' voices have been drowned out by the noise of the system. The only real way for them to be heard is through choice and competition. But our NHS generates an almost religious fervour, and resistance to reform is intense. A combination of strong commissioning, realistic tariffs, a broader financial base and effective regulation is needed to create an orderly market in which old and new providers can compete and thrive. Different providers can create unique services and provide real choice of care for cancer patients. Innovation in service delivery will require the creation of new clinics that can readily adopt novel technology. The existing model is simply unsustainable because of workforce shortages, de-motivation and top-down bureaucracy.

Getting the right treatment to the right patient using new diagnostics will increase the cost effectiveness of our care. Increased efficiency by the better use of expensive equipment, targeting expensive drugs to those that will really reap the benefits, and keeping patients out of hospital has to be part of our plan. We need to develop the excellent work of the major cancer charities, to make it easier for people to understand their treatment and make the best choices for themselves. Public, private and voluntary providers and payers working together have a vital role in developing innovative strategies to drive access, quality and value. Public education on healthy lifestyle change has never been more important to reduce the burden of disease.

It is essential that efficiency savings throughout cancer care delivery are ploughed back into service improvements. Our spending on new cancer drugs and high-quality radical radiotherapy is falling far behind comparable countries. Yet the per capita total amount spent on cancer is similar. Only by efficiency savings can funding be made available for innovation.

Over the next decade I believe we are going to continue to make tremendous strides in the treatment of cancer. It will become more prevalent throughout society as we all get older. But it will also become more treatable. As I said earlier, it will move from being a fatal to a chronic condition. Hopefully, as time goes on, it will become less chronic. Treatments will become less traumatic, and patients will be able to live for many years, with a high quality of life, even if their cancer is never completely cured.

But, as that happens, there will need to be a new compact between what I call the cancer industry, and between the patients. The industry – by which I mean doctors, clinical specialists, nurses, the drug companies and insurers – will need to become much more open with their patients. They should be honest with them, tell them about the range of treatments on offer, and explain how costs must be controlled. Too often the industry promises too much and delivers too little.

And patients should become more involved. Many are too passive, and too unwilling to take control of their own treatment. They expect everything to be done for them. But as cancer treatment develops, they will have to be partners in their own care. That means being realistic, and responsible, but also proactive.

Indeed, it may well be the case that the final breakthrough in that war on cancer I talked about earlier will not be a new drug, or a new type of surgery. It will be a change in the way cancer doctors and cancer patients work together.

This book, I hope, has been a modest but useful start in getting exactly this to happen.

Chapter Sixteen: Using the web wisely

There are over a billion sites on the web that are flagged up by searching for "cancer"

And the number is growing by the day. Frightening!

So how can you use the internet in the most constructive way to help yourself or someone you care for? Remember that most websites are there not to be helpful but to sell you something. It may be a product such as a book like this or a drug or an alternative medicine. It may be a service – a hospital or a clinic. Even charity websites want to sell you the charity as a good cause to get donations. Unfortunately, their marketing departments are more interested in your money than your health.

So, the first thing in approaching the web is to be completely cynical. A little harsh perhaps; but a very useful stance in which to go forward.

The second is not to get swamped with information from all sorts of dubious sites.

The third is that before you start surfing, ensure you have adequate information about exactly what your problem is. Ask for the pathology report and imaging results. Check what stage and grade the cancer is as described in this book. Make a small file to which you can constantly refer.

Then go to the top five sites first. If in Britain use the CancerResearchUK and MacMillan sites first. If you are in the US go to the National Cancer Institute and American Cancer Society sites in Washington.

Go to all of the "top six sites" listed below first and read about your cancer and its treatment in as much detail as possible. Then drill down to the disease specific sites. Go to some of the associated blogs where cancer patients chat about issues such as drug access and the availability of sophisticated types of radiotherapy.

Don't spend more than two hours surfing at each session or your brain will swell. Print out the key pieces of information for your file.

If you are computer savvy, keep online files – I'm just not that smart. Look at the linked sites – feel free to explore generally. Don't be put off by the medical terminology – google to clarify anything you don't understand.

If you want to look up academic papers on any cancer, go into Google Scholar. It gives you free access to a huge number of papers in the growing literature. They are sometimes very difficult to understand but if you persist you will crack the obtuse medical jargon. Do this especially if you are being offered a clinical trial or a new medication or procedure. All clinical trials can be easily found using a search engine and you will find far more detailed information than in many sanitised patient information leaflets. NHS websites are totally bland and patronizing and assume you are plain stupid. They don't explain rationing at all.

Try to build up a picture of your specific cancer, the diagnostic steps and the possible treatments. And go to the NICE website to check out their recommendations on what drugs and services should be available to cancer patients. Find out what other help is offered near where you live.

I've looked at all the websites below just before this book went to press. They all exist, and their address is correct. The top six are frequently updated – the others are variable. The sites often rely on a single person's enthusiasm and dedication. If they stop the site becomes inactive as they all require a lot of effort to maintain. There are many more helpful sites with local information. Ask around at your cancer centre, not just the doctors and nurses, but the reception staff and of course other patients. They will be a great source of local knowledge.

I leave you with just three thoughts to help you in your journey.

The first is to always interact pleasantly with all the healthcare staff you come across. Especially the underdogs in the system. They will all go the extra mile if they like you.

The second is to remember the young man in seat 20B. He acted within seconds – you can afford to take more time than he had to get out of the cancer maze, but you need to take charge of the situation. Only you can do it.

The third is to understand the importance and value of information: you need to become an informed patient. With information you can create a level playing field between you and your doctors. They won't be able to simply fob you off now.

Congratulations, you are now an 'empowered patient'. Good luck on your journey!

The top six
www.cancerresearchuk.org
Cancer Research UK. Very good, easy to read information on staging systems for each cancer and details of outcomes. Only read this bit if you really want to know the prognosis. Also contains a cancer help site. The most informative site on the technical aspects of cancer care and not too patronising.

www.macmillan.org.uk
The most informative UK site about services on offer to cancer patients. Stops short of telling you how to play the system like this book. Very good quality indeed.

www.cancer.org
A useful site from the American Cancer Society brimming with information on how to get better cancer care for yourself especially in the US. Essential reading.

http://www.nccn.org/patients/
A superb set of clinical care guidelines for all major cancers. Created and used by 32 leading cancer centres in the US it represents the gold standard of cancer care globally. Aspirational even for Britain!

https://www.nice.org.uk/guidance
The National Institute of Clinical Excellence is the final arbiter on what treatments the NHS will provide and pay for. You are hitting your head on a brick wall if you are trying to get a drug not approved for NHS use by NICE even though it may be available in all other European countries. You will need to use a different tack.

British sites
www.nhs.uk/cancer
The NHS lowdown on cancer. This site gives an overview of the disease, medicines and trials and a more in-depth A to Z of all the different types of cancer. Very politically correct, unlike this book. Tries hard to be friendly.

https://www.mariecurie.org.uk/help
Free UK nursing help. Marie Curie nurses help cancer patients retain quality of life and remain independent by offering free nursing care at home or in one of their hospices.

https://www.maggies.org/
A UK network of free, patient-focused centres. Maggie's 13 UK centres, one in Hong Kong and one in Barcelona bring emotional support, relaxation, information and practical advice. A little uncertain on its relationship to alternative medicine.

www.chaicancercare.org
Support for the UK's Jewish community. Chai provides free counselling, complementary therapies, advice and help with rights to services, centre-based rehabilitative and palliative care, group activities and home-based help. A truly excellent organisation.

www.cancerindex.org
A one-man-band guide to cancer on the internet by Simon Cotterill, a UK technology expert. His Guide to Internet Resources for Cancer aims to unscramble everything the web throws up and point patients towards the best sites under 12 helpful headings. A very interesting approach and a very useful mine of information.

www.canceractive.com
A patient-founded cancer charity which provides A to Z information on both conventional and complementary treatment and inspirational "survivor stories". A little alternative but otherwise very useful. A fun site generally.

www.fountaincentre.org
Support for patients at the Royal Surrey County Hospital. The Fountain Centre in the St Luke's unit of the hospital offers free complementary therapies and counselling and a programme of support groups.

www.wessexcancer.org.uk
Local support in six centres. The Wessex Cancer Trust offers onsite counselling and therapy, and information at its six support centres with two more underway. Financial grants and a holiday option are also available.

Specific cancers

Bladder cancer
www.actiononbladdercancer.org
A wealth of information and links to local support groups. Action on Bladder Cancer also shares personal stories and clinical trial data.

http://bladdercancersupport.org
Use the bladder cancer forum and access information on the American Bladder Cancer Society's website. There is also a Treatment Center Finder to quickly find the best services.

Blood and lymphatic cancers
www.leukaemiacare.org.uk
UK help for patients with blood and lymphatic cancers. Leukaemia CARE provides a 24 hour free phone service for people affected by leukaemia, Hodgkin, non-Hodgkin and other lymphomas, myeloma, myelodysplasia, myeloproliferative disorders and aplastic anaemia. There is a "speak to the nurse" and live chat options. The charity can also pair patients with a "phone buddy" volunteer for regular support.

www.lymphomas.org.uk
UK-based information and emotional support for patients with lymphatic cancers. The Lymphoma Association runs a free helpline, a series of support groups and a buddy scheme as well as online information and forums.

http://www.myeloma.org.uk/
Information and support for myeloma patients. Talk to a trained information specialist, meet other patients and read up on information and clinical trials.

Bone cancer
http://www.bcrt.org.uk/
Information, buddying and personal stories. The Bone Cancer Research Trust will match up patients with a volunteer within 48 hours. There is also information including on teenage cancers.

Brain tumours
www.braintumouraction.org.uk
UK-based emotional and practical support for brain tumour patients and families.

Brain Tumour Action provides a free helpline with trained counsellors, online support group, information and coordinates a UK network of face to face support groups.

www.braintumour.ca
Help for Canadians dealing with a brain tumour diagnosis. Family-founded Brain Tumour Foundation of Canada supplies a toll free phone line for one-to-one support, access to a network of adult and child brain tumour support groups, online networking and personal story posts. There is also a range of free publications available, including a family handbook.

www.btaa.org.au/
Patient led and focused website for brain tumour patients. A free Canadian handbook can be downloaded from Brain Tumour Alliance Australia. There is a freecall number, links to support groups as well as detailed information.

http://brainfoundation.org.au/
Brain tumour information. The Brain Foundation provides an A to Z of brain disorders and general information about brain tumours and cancers.

Breast cancer
www.breastcancercare.org.uk
UK support and information for patients with breast cancer. Breast Cancer Now runs a free support line, ask the nurse and forum plus easy to read information on breast cancer.

www.thehaven.org.uk
Free emotional, nutritional and physical support for women with breast cancer in the UK. The Haven operates six centres in England and Wales that guarantee each patient 10 free hours of therapy time and 2 hours with a specialist nurse. Family members can access free counselling. Each centre offers a programme of free or low cost classes, courses and talks. Other patients can phone the free helpline or watch video clips online.

www.breastcancergenetics.co.uk
National Helpline and support for people with breast cancer in the family. Provides personal stories from patients who have opted for preventative surgery. This is a complex area so don't be pressurized into family testing unless you are certain it's necessary.

www.bcna.org.au/
Get support for your breast cancer. Breast Cancer Network Australia gives women face-to-face group support or online networking. You can also read personal stories, download guides and fact sheets and access local services.

Gastrointestinal cancer
www.beatingbowelcancer.org
www.bowelcanceruk.org.uk
UK bowel cancer information. Another UK charity for patients with bowel cancer. Beating Bowel Cancer provides a low charge helpline with specialist nurses, email a nurse and online and local support groups as well as comprehensive information. Bowel Cancer UK's website has A to Z information about the disease including factsheets and statistics.

http://www.colorectal-cancer.ca/
Free information line and online support from the Colorectal Cancer Association of Canada. This includes access to "cancer coaches", support groups and guides to treatment and workplace issues.

https://www.pancreaticcancer.org.uk/
An excellent site from this charity. Full of helpful information and details of trials.

http://www.pancreaticcancercanada.ca/
Information-based support and a discussion forum. Pancreatic Cancer Canada also gives access to survivor stories and questions can be emailed to a medical doctor.

www.nostomachforcancer.org
Stomach cancer information and survivor stories. No Stomach for Cancer provides good information including hereditary facts, along with survivor stories, blogs and access to an online community. Also information about living without a stomach for those facing gastrectomy.

http://www.pancan.org
Free information, advice and support for US pancreatic cancer patients. Call Pancreatic Cancer Action Network's helpline for practical advice, search the clinical trial database, use the personalized medicine service and speak to a survivor or caregiver volunteer one-to-one, in a group or online.

Gynaecological cancer
www.jostrust.org.uk
UK-based information and support for women with cervical cancer. Jo's cervical runs a free helpline and provides an online resource kit. There is also an online forum, network of support groups and "ask the expert" panel for medical advice.

www.ovacome.org.uk
UK network for women with ovarian cancer. ovacome offers access to an online interactive support community, a free nurse-led helpline, and information and resources about the disease.

www.ovarian.org.uk
Information and personal experiences of ovarian cancer. Ovarian Cancer Action is a charity that funds research but also has information about ovarian cancer and a section where patients can read and share experiences.

www.ovariancanada.org
Free info, helpline and access to support groups. Ovarian Cancer Canada has a range of self-help guides, free phone support lines, teleconferences and information including on the latest clinical trial data.

www.ovariancancer.net.au
Great information and tools for women with ovarian cancer. Ovarian Cancer Australia gives you free online guides and tools for understanding and recording your cancer journey. There is support group info, questions and answers and personal stories.

http://www.nzgcf.org.nz/
Information and support on all gynaecological cancers. Gynaecological Cancer Foundation of New Zealand provides detailed guides, videos and a library and access to buddying and counselling.

Kidney cancer
https://www.kcuk.org.uk/
Kidney Cancer UK and the James Whale Fund have merged and are temporarily using this website for both. They provide detailed interactive UK information on kidney cancer including videos from kidney cancer experts. There is also a call line, a forum and "ask the nurse" and the Fund also awards grants to patients in economic hardship.

Lung cancer
www.roycastle.org
UK information and support for people with lung cancer. Roy Castle
Lung Cancer Foundation offers a free weekday helpline, detailed
information and access to support including a forum and help to stop
smoking.

www.lungcancercanada.ca
A wealth of information and support. Lung Cancer Canada offers
information, community events, a peer to peer network and clinical
trials data.

Prostate cancer
prostatecanceruk.org
The site of Prostate Cancer UK – Britain's leading prostate information
site.

Well validated and well set out with a specialist helpline, and local,
online, relationship, one to one and symptom support. Essential reading
for this disease especially with the new treatments emerging, which are
not likely to be approved by NICE [The National Institute for Health
and Care Excellence].

www.prostatecancersupport.org
Good guide to local support groups. Run by and for prostate cancer
patients and their families Prostate Cancer Support also mans a local
rate helpline run by trained volunteers.

https://zerocancer.org/
Support, help and info for US prostate cancer patients. Us TOO
International Prostate Cancer Education and Support Network gives
access to a toll free HelpLine, a network of support groups, and other
resources.

https://www.pcfa.org.au/
Detailed information and support groups. Prostate Cancer Foundation
of Australia as extensive information on its website from diagnosis to
research to living with the disease. You can also find out whether one of
the charity's specialist prostate cancer nurses is working near you.

https://prostate.org.nz/
A mix of information and support for the prostate cancer patient. The
Prostate Cancer Foundation provides peer support, an 0800 phone line

and information about prostate cancer.

http://prostatecancer.ca
Information about prostate cancer in Canada. Prostate Cancer Canada has collated all prostate cancer related information onto this easy-access site and also offers a free online and helpline Prostate Cancer Information Service.

Skin cancer
www.melanomauk.org.uk
Patient focused and patient run support group offering a freephone helpline and access to help with travel cost, information and patient stories.

https://www.melanoma.org.au/
Information and data, patient blogs and guides on skin cancer. The Melanoma Institute Australia runs a national network of researchers and clinicians based in Sydney at the Poche Centre.

Rare cancers
www.rarercancers.org.uk
UK support for patients with rarer cancers. The Rarer Cancers Foundation provides a free helpline, free patient interactive forum, patient stories and information. Very useful indeed if you have one of the uncommon cancers for which there is often little information.

Younger patients
www.youthcancertrust.org
Free holidays for young cancer patients. Youth Cancer Trust offers patients at UK hospitals aged between 14 and 30 free holidays in a Bournemouth guest house. Patients of the same age can also take part up to five years after treatment.

www.teenagecancertrust.org
Teenage only treatment units in the UK. Teenage Cancer Trust builds specialist treatment units within hospitals so teenage patients can be treated with their peers and by professionals skilled in this age group. Online, patients can create a facebook-style profile and there is also a network for family members.

http://childhoodcancer.ca
An oasis for families battling a child cancer diagnosis. The Childhood Cancer Foundation supplies a starter pack to families to help organise

and inspire them in their fight against the disease. A documentary on acute lymphoblastic leukemia, teen social networking, scholarships for young adult cancer survivors, and a benevolent fund for families in need of financial assistance are also available.

https://kidswithcancer.org.au/
Help for families struggling to pay for the costs of cancer. Kids with Cancer Foundation Australia funds families who are struggling financially with travel accommodation and grocery bills. There's no maximum per family per year, each application is reviewed on its own merit.

http://www.childcancer.org.nz/
A one stop shop for families of children with cancer. The Child Cancer Foundation provides broad-based support around hospital visits, a programme of activities, finance and a network to other families and other professionals.

Complementary and alternative medicine
www.cam-cancer.org
Scientific summaries of complementary and alternative medicine (CAM) efficacy for cancer. CAM-Cancer is an international project, launched by the European Commission, aimed at informing doctors and their patients.

www.pennybrohncancercare.org
All about UK complementary cancer care. The charity offers free information, courses at a dedicated centre in Bristol and a helpline on using complementary therapies and self-help techniques.

http://www.nhs.uk/Livewell/complementary-alternative-medicine/Pages/choose-CAM-practitioner.aspx
NHS guide to complementary therapies. Consult this for advice about how practitioners are regulated and links to approved practitioners.

Also published by *EER*

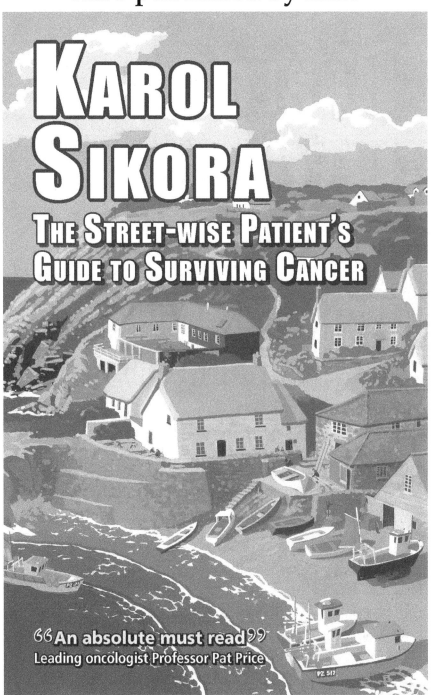

ROBERT LEFEVER

THE STREET-WISE GUIDE TO COPING WITH AND RECOVERING FROM ADDICTION

66 No one has ever written better about addiction. 99
– Jeffrey Robinson

GILL STEEL

THE STREET-WISE GUIDE
TO GETTING THE BEST FROM
YOUR LAWYER

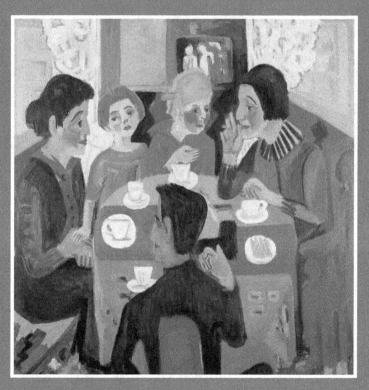

The Facey Romford Papers

DAYS IN THE LIFE OF THE NHS.
AN EVERYDAY STORY OF N£SD FOLK.

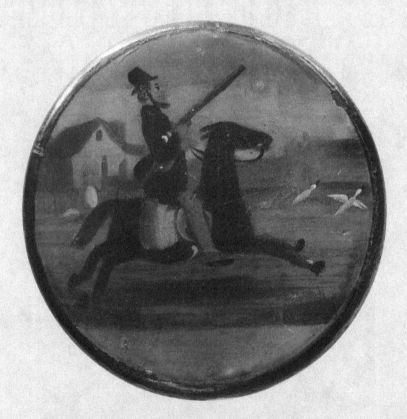

By Facey Romford, Jr

With a Preface by Roy Lilley

'COMING, READY OR NOT!'

The Realities, the Politics, and the Future of the NHS

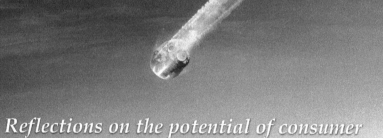

Reflections on the potential of consumer power to renovate health care.

John Spiers

Foreword by Philip Booth